INDUSTRIAL TOXICOLOGY AND DERMATOLOGY IN THE PRODUCTION AND PROCESSING OF PLASTICS

ELSEVIER MONOGRAPHS ON TOXIC AGENTS

Edited by

ETHEL BROWNING, M.D.

FORMERLY H.M. MEDICAL INSPECTOR OF FACTORIES,
MINISTRY OF LABOUR AND NATIONAL SERVICE,
LONDON (GREAT BRITAIN)

ELSEVIER PUBLISHING COMPANY
AMSTERDAM – LONDON – NEW YORK

INDUSTRIAL TOXICOLOGY AND DERMATOLOGY IN THE PRODUCTION AND PROCESSING OF PLASTICS

by

K. E. MALTEN

LECTURER IN OCCUPATIONAL DERMATOLOGY,
ROMAN CATHOLIC UNIVERSITY,
NIJMEGEN (THE NETHERLANDS)

and

R. L. ZIELHUIS

OCCUPATIONAL PHYSICIAN, NETHERLANDS
INSTITUTE FOR PREVENTIVE MEDICINE,
LEIDEN (THE NETHERLANDS)

ELSEVIER PUBLISHING COMPANY
AMSTERDAM – LONDON – NEW YORK
1964

SOLE DISTRIBUTORS FOR THE UNITED STATES AND CANADA
AMERICAN ELSEVIER PUBLISHING COMPANY, INC.
52 VANDERBILT AVENUE, NEW YORK 17, N.Y.

SOLE DISTRIBUTORS FOR GREAT BRITAIN
ELSEVIER PUBLISHING COMPANY LIMITED
12B, RIPPLESIDE COMMERCIAL ESTATE
RIPPLE ROAD, BARKING, ESSEX

LIBRARY OF CONGRESS CATALOG CARD NUMBER 63-11368

WITH 6 ILLUSTRATIONS AND 8 TABLES

'And quickly as we see wines flow through a strainer, sluggish oil on the other hand is slow to do so, because sure enough it consists of elements either larger in size or more hooked and tangled in one another.

Again things which look to us hard and dense must consist of particles more hooked together, and be held in union because all welded through with branch-like elements.'

LUCRETIUS
Roman poet and philosopher
96 (?)–55 B.C.
in: *De Rerum Natura*

(P. C. RITCHIE, *A Chemistry of Plastics and High Polymers*, Cleaver-Hume, London, 1949)

Preface

To think of modern every day life without plastics has become unimaginable. Plastics have penetrated into every field of industrial production or scientific work thanks to the adaptability of these materials to nearly every purpose of use.

Variation in synthesis makes it possible to combine properties which in former years were separated over a number of classical materials. Moreover they offer possibilities of connecting various classical materials in a hitherto unforeseen way, for instance the junction of ceramics to metals. Thus plastics are more than simple substitutes for classical materials and they therefore will be produced and applied to an ever-increasing degree.

In old times, plastics were made of naturally occurring substances, which were modified in one way or another to yield a new product adapted more or less to the purpose for which it should be used, for instance oilskin, derivatives of cellulose, natural rubber, proteins and so on. These are not under consideration in this book. The industrial-hygienic properties of synthetic rubbers have very ably been discussed by Schultheiss (1959). We do not think it appropriate to reduplicate this field.

We wish to discuss only the entirely synthetized plastics: a long range of completely new materials which began in 1902 with the synthesis of Novolaks, followed by Bakelites in 1907, Albertols in 1910, the vinyl compounds in 1912 and the urea resins in 1918 up to the newest development in the field of silicones and poly-urethanes.

At the moment articles of every day use made of these materials are put into the hand of consumers, they are generally entirely harmless: every manufacturer will always try by all means possible to produce innocuous end-products ready for appropriate use. But as soon as intermediate products are delivered, which can be applied and processed upon by lay-men or in small workshops, for instance glues, paints, stoppers, textile finishes, care should be taken with a number of them. The same is true of manufactured moulding: a certain group of plastics may show untoward effects if they are not handled in the prescribed way.

These untoward effects are far from frequent and a great number of manufacturers have never had any complaints in their mills. The materials they handle and their methods of processing never reach toxicological or dermatological literature. In a relatively small number of cases, however, untoward effects are seen, and it is the purpose of this book to point to these exceptions and to describe the methods of preventing them.

Although it has been written especially for industrial medical officers, we hope that a wider public may also find some items of interest. To the latter group we wish to underline that we are not hoisting the stormflag: in everybody's work there is a hidden or evident risk; for example, coalminers or seamen or space aviators. But it is our duty to minimize these risks in order to be able to build a world in which there is a place in the sun for everybody.

The survey presented in this book will undoubtedly be incomplete. New hazards may exist, which have not yet found their way into the literature covered by us. Some of the risks described will perhaps refer to procedures already out of date. The authors would appreciate very much any information of additional experiences of toxicological and dermatological risks, either not covered in this book or not reviewed adequately.

Confrontation of the authors with industrial-hygienic aspects of plastics took place for the greater part in their past (M) and present (Z) work in the Department for Occupational Medicine of the Netherlands Institute for Preventive Medicine at Leiden and in the Dermatological Department of the R.C. University of Nijmegen (M).

We thank the Directors and the Governing Board of these Institutes for the opportunity given to us to study this interesting field and for the permission to publish this book. We also wish to acknowledge the help of Mr. P. A. Reitsma in reviewing the techno-chemical part of this work, the assistance of Mrs. N. K. J. Arps-Hill in reviewing the translation and of Mrs. E. Snethlage in documentation work. Moreover we want to thank the directors of mills in which personal observations were made, and the workmen who cooperated for this purpose.

Last but not least we are greatly indebted to the numerous authors who committed their experiences to paper, surely mainly in their 'spare time', and to an ever increasing number of producers of intermediate or auxiliary substances with trade names, who provided us with the exact chemical compounding of their products. We want to emphasize that without such information it would be impossible to undertake investigations with the purpose of eliminating harmful effects to our fellowmen.

The schemes are drawn and the photographs are taken by the Department of Medical Illustration of the R. C. University of Nijmegen.

Nijmegen/Leiden
October 1963

K. E. Malten
R. L. Zielhuis

Contents

1

Chemical composition and biological activity

DEFINITIONS

A plastic is a substance essentially constituted of organic *macromolecules*. For moulding purposes it is processed under conditions in which it is, or can be made, transformable. Under usage conditions it appears stable and keeps the shape which has been given to it during moulding.

The term *resin* is used to denote all medium- or high-molecular intermediate substances (their eventual content of modifiers excluded), from which plastics are made. The term *plastics* is used for all industrial end products ready for every day use (including glues etc., which are intermediates) or as a material to replace classical materials, as for instance plastic foils to replace leather or textile goods, plastic plates to replace wood, veneer or glass plates or metal sheets, and which, like the classical materials, may be processed further in the classical ways, *e.g.* by sawing, filing, lathing or glueing.

An enormous number of one type of organic micromolecules, or of a restricted number of different ones, are linked together to form a macromolecule. Thus, generally, the macromolecule roughly shows the same empirical formula as the constituting micromolecules. Setting aside that the macromolecular chains may be terminated by a pair of monovalent groupings, which differ from the monomer structure (for instance derived from the solvent employed), macromolecules made by *polymeri-*

References p. 20

zation indeed have the same empirical formula as have the monomers. In the macromolecules made by *polycondensation* the atomic composition differs from the sum of the empirical formulae of the constituting basic materials in forming byproducts, which are excluded from the same reaction.

PRINCIPLES OF CHEMICAL SYNTHESIS

Two principal synthetic procedures must be distinguished: polymerization and polycondensation.

Polymerization

The macromolecules are built up from numerous uniform units: *the monomers* (which are the molecular structure elements for the polymer end products). No byproducts are formed. An opening of unsaturated intermolecular bonds in the monomers almost always underlies this kind of reaction. Once initiated, it proceeds like an avalanche towards the high polymer end products.

A=A	+	A=A	→ –A–A–A–A–	Homopolymerization
A=A	+	B=B	→ –A–A–B–B–	Copolymerization
A=A	+	C	→ –A–A–C–A–A –	Heteropolymerization

As the whole chemical process of polymerization (setting aside the chemical properties of the monomer molecule) is highly dependable upon factors such as temperature, pressure, kinds of solvents, catalysts, inhibitors, chain-transferring materials and impurities, in industrial practice the whole process is executed in a closed system until the fully polymerized substance ensues. An exception to this 'rule' is provided by the curing of unsaturated polyesters (see p. 72).

With respect to the theoretical background of the polymerization reaction the following brief remarks may be made:

The C-atoms next to a saturated bond are linked together by

a so-called homopolar bond consisting of two shared electrons. An unsaturated bond consists, besides the normal homopolar bond, of a second pair of shared electrons, which are present in a somewhat more exposed position. These are called π-electrons. On the one hand, the double bond is stronger than the single one, on the other hand, it shows a greater reactivity due to the more exposed position of the π-electrons. Free *radicals* (if not stabilized through special possibilities of resonance) are extremely reactive atoms or molecules characterized by an unpaired electron.

The action of a phenyl radical upon an unsaturated C=C bond can be represented as follows: the radical attracts that one of the two π-electrons which has an opposite spin to its own unpaired electron, and in this way a new homopolar bond, consisting of two shared electrons arises between the radical and the C=C structure. The second π-electron is repelled to the other side of the radical–monomer combination, thus giving rise to a new radical function: monomer radical. This monomer radical will repeat the same sequence of events with another monomer, immediately giving rise to a dimer radical and so on, until-high polymer radicals are formed.

From the above it becomes clear that 3 phases may be discerned:

1. *Initiation:* the formation of free radicals from a radical-donor structure, usually called *catalyst*, starter or initiator. In the case of benzoylperoxide initiation may occur by augmentation of temperature or adding a cobalt compound (which may be called *accelerator)*.

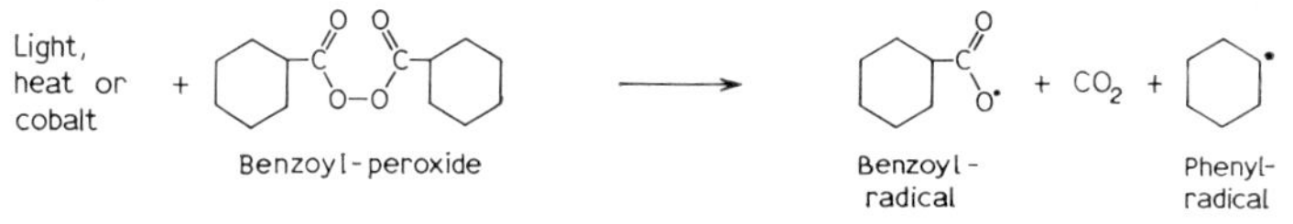

2. *Propagation:* the chain reaction following upon reaction of

the radical with a monomer thus forming a monomer radical, which acts in the same way with another monomer encountered.

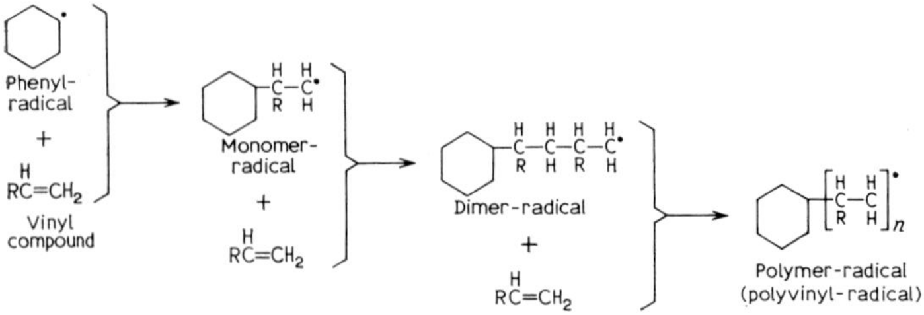

3. *Termination:*

a. The polymer radical meets another radical with which it reacts under formation of a saturated (homopolar) bond; this may occur with a catalyst radical or with another polymer radical.

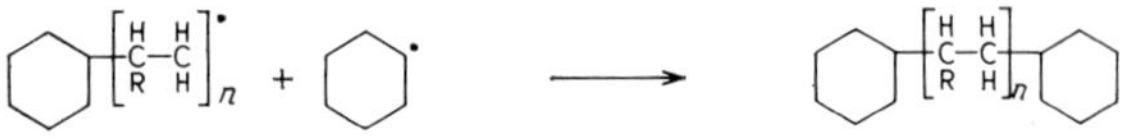

b. The polymer radical meets another monomer from which a hydrogen atom is withdrawn under formation of a new radical from the unsaturated monomer, which starts a new polymerization chain reaction (chain transfer).

$$\sim\!\sim CHR-CH_2-CHR-CH_2\cdot \; + \; CHR=CH_2 \; \rightarrow$$
$$\sim\!\sim CHR-CH_2-CHR-CH_3 \; + \; CH_2=CR\cdot$$

c. The polymer radical combines with a solvent molecule in a chain-transfer reaction by which parts of the solvent molecule are built in as a final group in the polymer and a new radical originating from the solvent is formed.

$$\sim\!\sim CHR-CH_2\cdot \; + \; CCl_4 \; \rightarrow \; \sim\!\sim CHR-CH_2-CCl_3 \; + \; Cl\cdot$$

Chain transfer always means lowering the degree of polymerization (= the number of monomers per macromolecule). In practice this principle is often used to confine the degree of polymerization to a certain average level by adding substances which promote chain transfer (this is a kind of modifier, see below).

The polymerization reaction initiated in a few centers continues like an avalanche, until all available monomers have taken part in the propagation reaction; intermediate, semicured compounds are not formed, nor are byproducts. *Grosso modo*, the polymerization end-product has the same percentual distribution of atoms as the monomer, except the now saturated head-and-tail configurations which may be derived from the catalyst or from the solvent. Numerically these head-and-tail configurations are insignificant, except in cases of frequent chain transfer with solvent molecules (in which case moreover solvent radicals are formed, which physiologically may not be inert) or if too much catalyst is present, giving rise to a great number of short chains. Technically both circumstances will be avoided because they lead to inappropriate short-chained end-products, whereas high-molecular end-products are the industrial goal. But in experimental production or in case of technical troubles both possibilities should be borne in mind, because they may give rise to untoward biological effects. In industrial practice, however, *the polymerization end-products hardly contain any active functional groups* or residues of low-molecular substances, which were necessary for initiation or as a milieu in which the propagation reaction could develop. Moreover, these low-molecular substances are washed out after termination (as far as they are not occluded by the high-molecular particles) to obtain a purified polymerization end-product which is usually in the form of a powder or granules. During moulding, this fully polymerized product is made viscous again by heating. Modifiers (stabilizers, plasticizers, colours etc.) may be mixed through the viscous material after which the mixture is set in the desired shape by cooling. Thus, moulding and setting of polymerizates is an entirely *physical process*. Possibility of con-

References p. 20

tact with highly active intermediate polymerization substances does not occur provided the closed system remains intact. Only just before and during moulding, there is a possibility of biological contact with modifiers. After setting, the final product may be machined.

The *tendency to polymerization* depends on several factors: The tendency is higher, the more the electrical polarity of the monomers is raised. Isobutylene for instance has a greater polarity than butylene.

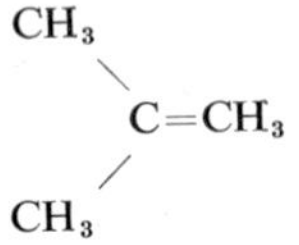

Isobutylene

$$CH_3-CH=CH-CH_3$$

Butylene

Substitution may change the polarity or may cause an effect of sterical hindrance. Conjugated double bonds (alternating saturated and unsaturated bonds) may more easily be activated than isolated double bonds (two or more saturated bonds between the unsaturated ones).

The following types of polymerization may be distinguished:

a. isopolymerization = homopolymerization: only one kind of monomer takes part in the process. Examples: polyethylene, polyvinylchloride, polystyrene.

b. copolymerization: different kinds of monomers, each of which is itself capable of polymerization, take part in the process. Examples: Buna-S (butadiene plus styrene monomers), polyvinylchloride–acetate (vinylchloride plus vinylacetate monomers).

c. heteropolymerization: one of the monomers or reactants is not capable of polymerization but it becomes activated by another kind of monomer which in itself is capable of polymerization. Example: maleic acid plus styrene monomer.

A special kind of heteropolymerization is called *poly-addition:* two different monomers, each of which is not capable of polymerization, react by exchange of atoms or atom groups and thus may form high-polymer products. The mechanism of this reaction is different from the simple polymerization. Examples: polyurethanes (see p. 85) and ethoxylin resins (= epoxy resins), (see p. 104).

In practice, the following procedures are known:

1. *Block polymerization*: the whole process is executed with the reactants as such without the aid of solvents or diluents.
2. *Polymerization in a fluid milieu* which may be a solvent of the mono- and eventually also of the polymer, or a non-solvent of the mono- and polymer: suspension polymerization and emulsion polymerization.
3. *Polymerization in the gaseous phase.*
4. *Aerosol polymerization*: nebulizing the dissolved monomer in a gaseous catalyst.

The choice of procedure depends on the properties of the monomers, on the desired usage properties of the end-product, on the catalysts and on the possibility of conveying the heat of the exothermic reaction.

Polycondensation

Two molecules are said to condense, when they unite by mutual elimination of a small simple molecule such as H_2O or R–OH, each condensing molecule contributing a portion of the eliminated molecule (= byproduct, which is excluded from building the final polycondensate). (Exception: caprolactam, see p. 186 and unsaturated polyesters, p. 71).

Polycondensation reactions are equilibrium reactions, that is to say, they proceed only if the byproduct is taken away from the mixture of reactants.

In contrast to the polymerization process, in polycondensation the growing capacity of the newly formed molecules

References p. 20

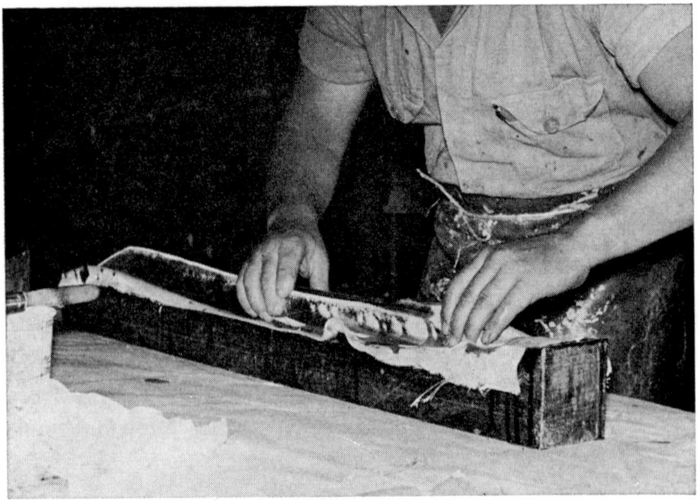

Fig. 1. Hand lay-up method. Glass-fibre cloth with epoxy resin hardener mixture.

decreases with increasing length, and the polycondensation process starts multicentrically. Both these peculiarities cause the formation of many low-molecular chains. The properties of the medium- or high-molecular end-product depend on the properties of the original reactants, their mutual concentrations, the temperature, the kinds of catalysts or solvents eventually used.

It is possible to stop the polycondensation reaction at any desired moment: a mixture of medium-molecular compounds, each with a number of chemically active groups results. Such a mixture of low- and medium-molecular compounds is called an *intermediate* product or *semicured* resin. It can generally be stored for some time in a viscous semisolid or even solid state as raw material, and mailed to the manufacturer of plastic articles. It may further be processed by pressing and/or heating the mass in a mould of the desired shape and either starting the polycondensation reaction again or starting a cross-linking reaction, both leading by further chemical reaction to the desired high-molecular end-product. For re-initiation purposes heating, or adding *catalysts* (= hardeners = curing agents) is necessary.

Modifiers such as pigments, fillers, antimould agents, plasticizers, etc. may be added in the first stage or in the second (= curing) stage of the above-mentioned reactions.

This second stage, by which an intermediate product is given its final shape, is called the *curing* of the plastic.

As an example of a polycondensation reaction the two-step condensation of a phenolformaldehyde plastic may be given: the first step in acid medium leading to the linear phenoplast (an intermediate product), and the second step in alkaline medium after adding surplus formaldehyde, finally leading to the formation of the cured end-product.

Step 1

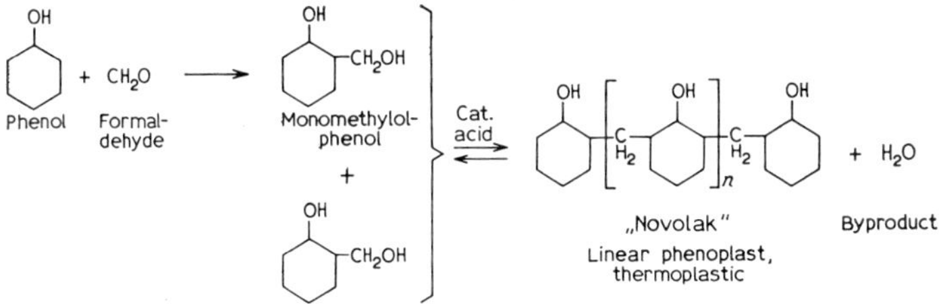

Step 2

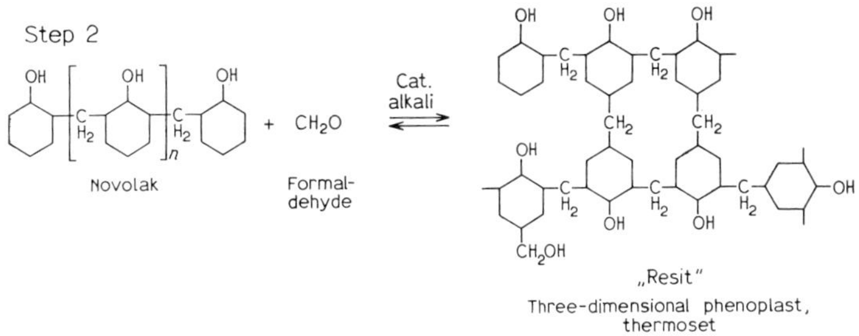

The possibility of interruption and chemically restarting the polycondensation reaction at any desired moment invites one to apply rather simple moulding procedures (hand-lay-up-methods) involving as a consequence great possibilities of biological contact with semicured, chemically still very active resins and all the other low-molecular added substances (modifiers), particularly with curing agents and catalysts. The curing of condensates is a *chemical process*.

BIOLOGICAL HAZARD

In practice, an unwritten law seems to hold true: the larger the macromolecules, the less they are chemically and physically active. We are inclined to add: the less they are active from a toxicological or sensitizing point of view (carcinogenesis after foil implantations being excluded).

Thus, in polymerization processes alertness is necessary in handling some of the monomers and the very sporadically occurring low polymers; the polymerization end-products, being high-molecular during moulding, need less attention.

This is in sharp contrast with polycondensation: a number of basic components of polycondensation resins and the incompletely cured condensates (or uncombined components therein) may be the causes of untoward effects, apparently partly related to their low molecularity, because fully cured polycondensates are usually also inert. A second contrast is that the catalyst of polymerization is added in the *closed*-system phase (exception see p. 72) and occluded in the end-product or washed out before moulding, whereas in polycondensation catalysts or curing agents are openly added to the semicured resins (usually in surplus quantities). Polyaddition reactions may also take place in open systems. The third contrast concerns *moulding:* a mechanized physical process in polymerization, but in polycondensation a chemical process, which is executed during intimate biological contact due to the frequent use of rather simple processing methods (hand-lay-up), and from which may emanate a low-molecular active byproduct (for instance formaldehyde).

Mostly the end-products of simple polymerization do not possess the properties necessary for usage. By the addition of usually low-molecular substances, the end-products can be better adapted to usage conditions. In polymerization plastics, these *modifying substances* are added after termination of the whole polymerization process: they are incorporated during the physical process of moulding. In order to make a polymerization plastic mouldable, it must be made viscous by heating. The heat generally obviates manual contact with the mixture of polymerizate and modifiers. In polycondensation plastics too the modifiers, if used, are added just before moulding. At this phase the biologically active intermediate polycondensation substances are usually in a liquid or semiliquid state of moderate temperature. Thus there is a risk of handling both these groups of materials during mixing. If, moreover, a cold-curing process is used, there may be additional opportunity for close biological contact during moulding (hand-lay-up method). If, however, only heat is used for the curing of the intermediate polycondensate, further contact with low- and medium-molecular substances and modifiers may be obviated by the temperature. These modifying substances used in both kinds of plastics may also be sensitizers or irritants, but apparently seldom act as such.

Two pitfalls should be mentioned here, both of which are more or less theoretical. A number of plasticizers (see Chapter 3) are not only solvents for resinous compounds, but also for added modifying substances which may be present in such low concentrations that their toxicity may be disregarded (*e.g.* stabilizers). When thermoplastic end products are further processed by locally applied heat or pressure for the manufacturing of commodities, a fairly large quantity of plasticizers may migrate to the surface, carrying with it a considerable quantity of the stabilizer. Thus, *e.g.*, girls welding thermoplastic sheets into

References p. 20

portfolios can be exposed to a larger quantity of the stabilizer than would seem likely. The second pitfall that should not be overlooked is that impurities in any of the ingredients used, *e.g.* naphthalenes in phthalic acid anhydride (see p. 67) may cause untoward effects.

Finally, one remark should be made: in plastics, when subjected to unusual, unforeseen conditions, or simply through ageing, *degradation (decomposition)* of the high-molecular compounds may occur, releasing the original monomers or new disintegration products of biologically active low-molecular composition. Phenoplasts may decompose into phenol, benzene, toluene, cresol and other aromatic hydrocarbons; polyesters disintegrate into acids and alcohols. Moreover, added low-molecular modifying substances may migrate under 'special' circumstances (tricresylphosphate poisoning of butter kept in a plastic butter dish!). Both circumstances indicate that the rule that cured-out plastics are harmless materials is not a hard and fast one.

2

Thermoplasts and thermosetting resins

If a material is softened by the application of heat, so that it can be moulded, and hardens again on cooling, and if this process can be repeated indefinitely, the material is described as thermoplastic. *Thermoplasts* are *linear* macromolecules, *e.g.* polyvinylchloride, polyethylene.

If, on the other hand, the material softens on heating, but can on continued application of heat be converted into a rigid product, which is no longer softened by further heating, it is classified as *thermohardening* or *thermosetting*. During heating a chemical reaction takes place by which macromolecules are linked together to form network structures. Network structures can also be obtained in a cold-curing process in which macromolecules are linked together by means of the added curing agent: in this case the heat is not applied externally but generated internally in the chemical reaction.

Whether linear macromolecules or network structures are formed depends on the functionality of the reactants. By functionality is meant the number of valencies in a certain compound capable of reacting under certain circumstances. Basic materials can be classified with respect to the number of functions *(f)* they bear.

Two-dimensional (= linear) products result from reaction between two substances each bearing 2 functions (so-called 2:2 reactions). The reaction product also possesses 2 functions

References p. 20

Methanol	$H_3\overset{*}{C}$—OH	$f = 1$
Vinylchloride	$H_2\overset{*}{C}{=}\overset{*}{C}HCl$	$f = 2$
Formaldehyde	$H_2\overset{*}{\underset{*}{C}}{=}O$	$f = 2$
Glycerol	$H_2\overset{*}{C}$—OH | HC*—OH | $H_2\underset{*}{C}$—OH	$f = 3$

which in turn can produce the same reaction, thus forming high-polymer linear structures. Examples are:

(a) 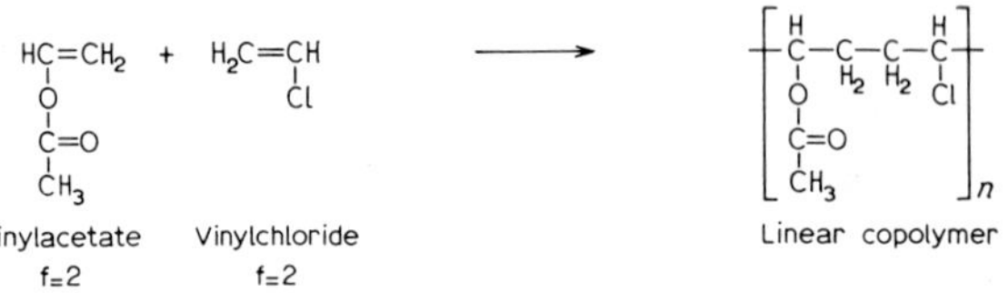

(b) 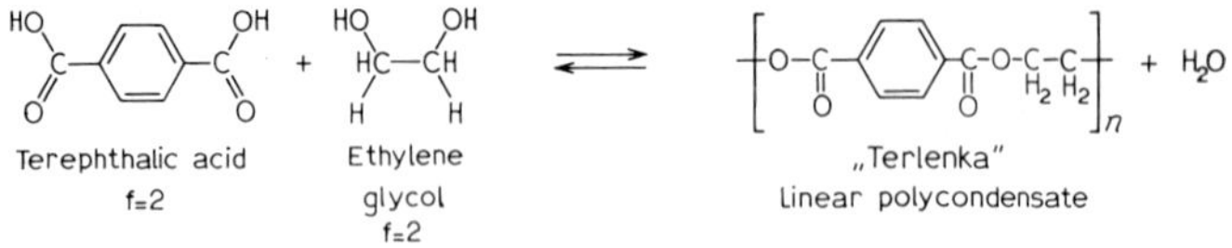

Three-dimensional network structures result if one of the reactants has 2 functions and the other carries at least 3 functions (2 : 3 reactions), *e.g.* polyesters (see next page).

The number of active functions in a molecule is dependent on the circumstances under which the reaction takes place: for instance phenol and formaldehyde condense into linear poly-

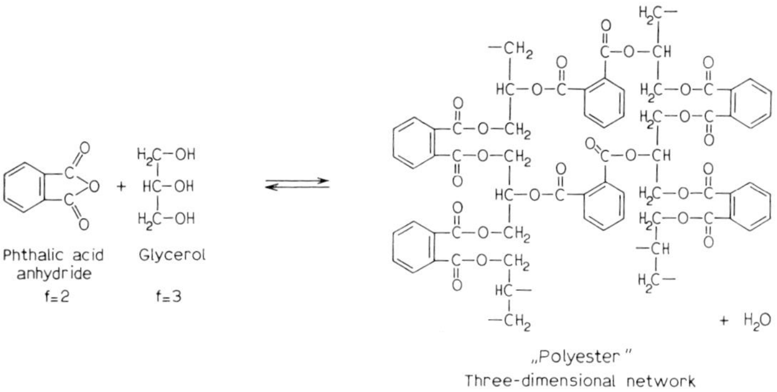

condensates in an acid medium (2:2 reaction), but in an alkaline medium phenol carries 3 functions (3:2 reaction) and thus a three-dimensional network will be formed. Aniline and formaldehyde react according to a 2:2 reaction in a medium of low acidity and to a 3:2 reaction in a medium of high acidity.

From the laws of functionality it may be seen that polymerization does not always result in thermoplastic resins: polyethylene can normally be considered a thermoplastic, but it can be crosslinked (polymerization) with peroxide to give a thermoset material. On the other hand, polycondensation does not always lead to thermosetting resins (see above: Terlenka). Sometimes materials are made by applying both principles successively: linear unsaturated polyesters (made themselves by polycondensation) may be cured by adding unsaturated crosslinking agents, for instance styrene, leading via heteropolymerization to high-molecular network end-products (see p. 72).

Thus, if the linear macromolecules are large enough, that is to say at the moment the Van der Waals forces reach a certain level, the linear macromolecular substance will appear as a solid under usage conditions (thermoplastic). Only when the macromolecules are linked together (three-dimensional network) a thermosetting material may ensue.

3

Auxiliary substances

In processing plastics or in adapting the end-products to special requirements of use a great number of auxiliary substances are used. A number of these substances are grouped here under a few headings. If untoward effects of these substances are known, these are fully enumerated in the various chapters.

a. Catalysts

In former years, a catalyst was defined as a substance which influenced the reaction velocity, but could be recovered as such after the reaction had occurred. In the field of plastics, however, most of the catalysts are finally incorporated in the end-product. Catalysts used in polycondensation (*e.g.* alkalies and acids) are generally less aggressive than those used in polymerization (*e.g.* organic peroxides, boranes, aluminium-alkyl compounds).

b. Inhibitors

retard the polymerization reaction because, for instance, they immediately react with the free radicals unintentionally originating from peroxidic catalysts (*e.g.* phenols, diamines, picric acid).

c. Accelerators

speed up the formation of free radicals from the catalysts (*e.g.* cobalt naphthenate promotes the formation of peroxide radicals). These substances need only be present in small quantities and are generally bound in the polymerization end-products.

d. Stabilizers

impede spontaneous polymerization (*e.g.* hydroquinone added to styrene) or degradation of the polymers. With regard to degradation of the polymers the following may be said. When a vinylchloride polymer is subjected to heat or light, two degradation reactions occur:

1. *Heat degradation* which causes loss of hydrogen chloride, thus forming conjugated double bond structures (which are chromophoric) and at the same time oxidation of these polyene systems probably gives rise to carbonyl groups. Stabilizers act through removing free hydrogen chloride.

2. *Photo-degradation.* When polymers are exposed to light, oxidation (leading to chain scission and cross-linkage) seems to be the main cause of breakdown. In light stabilization there seems to be a trend towards the use of ultraviolet absorbers to eliminate certain wavelengths that cause the degradations (*e.g.* phenyl salicylate (Salol), 2,4-dihydroxybenzophenone (Uvinol 400), 2,2-dihydroxy-4-methoxybenzophenone). Other light stabilizers act in a different way that cannot be explained by a single mechanism. Of dominant significance may be the free-radical mechanism; this means that the stabilizing chemical reacts with the polymer radical formed by a previous extraction of a hydrogen atom from the polymer. The stabilizing chemical thus prevents an autocatalytic action by blocking further cross-linking and oxidation reactions at this particular point. Light stabilizers are, *e.g.*, dibutyl-tin dilaureate, epoxidized oils, barium–cadmium systems.

e. Antioxidants

are compounds which counteract atmospheric (photo-) oxidation of unsaturated double bonds (*e.g.* hydroquinone derivatives, phenols, amines, oximes, dilaurylthiodipropionate).

f. Antistatics

prevent accumulation of static electricity. This aim may be

References p. 20

reached by admixture of substances conducting electricity themselves or indirectly by absorbing water. The latter always show an oleophilic group (for compatibility with polymer resins) and a hydrophilic, or better: a hygroscopic group (for conductance of electricity), *e.g.* stannochloride, MoS_2, cetylalcohol. Another way by which the aim is reached is a surface treatment of end-products with chemicals, again being at one side oleophilic and at the other side hydrophilic, *e.g.* several types of detergents.

g. Foaming agents

cause the sponge structure by releasing vapour or gas during setting of the plastic (*e.g.* azoisobutyronitrile, ammonium carbonate, chlorinated hydrocarbons).

h. Lubricants

are non-wetting, non-swelling, non-volatile substances which, interposed between the linear macromolecules, increase their mutual distance and therefore decrease the intermolecular binding capacities (Van der Waals forces); they are only in small quantities compatible with polymer resins (*e.g.* calcium stearate, polyethylene wax). They increase extensibility.

i. Plasticizers

are high-boiling organic compounds (usually liquids), which act as solvents for resinous substances. The incorporation of plasticizers into polymers reduces the secondary attractive forces (Van der Waals forces) between the polymer chains, thereby rendering the polymer substance softer, more flexible and easier to process. Such an organic compound must possess high compatibility with the resin, so that a sufficient amount of the plastifying compound can be incorporated to give exactly the desired mechanical property to the plasticized polymer. To be effective, a plasticizer must be a substance which is sufficiently attracted (polar) to the polymer unions to be able to insert itself between these secondary bonds and replace them by polymer–plasticizer–polymer linkages. It is customary to classify plasticizers as primary and secondary plasticizers, and as extenders. The primary types exhibit high solvency or good compatibility with the resin and may be used alone as plasticizers. The secondary plasticizers are poor solvents and in most cases cannot be used alone as plasticizers. Nonetheless, the role of the secondary plasticizers is important since many desirable properties, such as low-temperature flexibility, ageing stability, non-inflammability can be realized through their judicious use. The extenders are virtually non-solvents for the polymer and are used to reduce the costs of a particular formulation or compound. The most important primary plasticizers are the phthalate esters, such as dibutylphthalate and di-ethylhexylphthalate. Also important are polybasic acid esters: *e.g.* the dialkyl esters of adipic or sebacic acid (giving extremely low temperature flexibility); polymeric plasticizers: *e.g.* polyethylene glycol (finding use as plasticizer for proteins, casein and polyvinyl alcohol); further substances of the polyester type, *i.e.* saturated dibasic acids, esterified with glycols and terminated with monobasic acids. While the polyester-type plasticizers are seldom used alone, such properties as resistance to migration, resistance to extraction by gasoline, oil, water, soap, detergents, as well as low volatility are realized in combination with monomeric plasticizers in, *e.g.*, polyvinyl chloride formulations. Halogenated hydrocarbons (paraffinic and aromatic) are considered secondary plasticizers, *e.g.* chlorinated paraffins are compatible with vinyl chloride-type resin.

j. Fillers

may be added in large amounts, not only to economize the use of the plastic but also to confer various new properties to the end-products, for instance a lessened inflammability or an increased abrasion resistance. Well known are amorphous silicium dioxide, lithopone, chalk, wood products, etc.

References p. 20

k. Solvents

are very important as milieu factors in which polymerization occurs. A great number of organic substances may be applied, *e.g.*, toluene, benzene, amyl acetate, ethyl acetate. Their biological acitivity is generally well described in toxicological textbooks. A few are used more or less specifically in the processing of various plastics and they will be discussed together under their specific headings.

l. Colorants

available for colouring plastics are:

Dyes, which are synthetic or natural organic chemicals, soluble in most common solvents; they are transparent, *e.g.*, nigrosine.

Pigments, organic and inorganic types being used; they are mostly opaque and not soluble, *e.g.*, titanium dioxide, iron oxide, chrome yellow, ultramarine blue.

m. Antimould agents

such as tricresyl phosphate, tetramethylthiuram disulfide, stearates of Ca, Zn, Al.

REFERENCES

(Chapters 1, 2 and 3)

Many technical books and magazines give introductory papers regarding the chemistry of plastics. The authors chiefly made use of the following.

HERMANS, P. H., *Inleiding tot de Theoretische Organische Chemie*, Elsevier, Amsterdam, 1952.

RITCHIE, P. D., *A Chemistry of Plastics and High Polymers*, Cleaver, London, 1949.

RUNGE, F., *Einführung in die Chemie und Technologie der Kunststoffe*, Akademischer Verlag, Berlin, 1959.

SCHAEFER, W., *Einführung in das Kunststoffgebiet*, Geest & Portig, Leipzig, 1953.

4

Occupational diseases of the skin in the plastics industry

DEFINITION AND CRITERIA FOR DIAGNOSIS

An occupational dermatosis can be defined as 'a pathological condition of the skin for which occupational exposure can be shown to be a major causal or contributory factor' (Lane 1942). With a few exceptions, the skin diseases which are encountered as a result of industrial exposure do not vary significantly from those encountered in non-industrial practice. In order to recognize a certain skin ailment as an industrial dermatosis a number of criteria should be fulfilled as far as possible:

a. The patient must have been in contact with the incriminated noxa in his work.

b. The lapse of time between the exposure and the onset of the dermatosis must be in accordance with the type of the particular noxious influence and with the clinical phenomena.

c. Generally the first symptoms must have appeared at the site of maximal exposure.

d. The observed skin anomalies must be similar to those which may be encountered in workers exposed to the same noxious influence in similar jobs.

e. Non-occupational exposure should not have occurred.

f. Careful analysis must show improvement after interruption of the work contact and recurrence of the symptoms on resumption of the incriminated work.

References p. 39

g. If skin function tests for particular skin diseases are practicable, they should confirm the expectation.

These criteria must be handled carefully and with great skill, because some occupational skin diseases normally show exceptions to these rules (see for instance: localization in allergic contact-type eczematous dermatitis).

PRIMARY IRRITATION *versus* ALLERGIC SENSITIZATION

Apart from a host of rare occupational skin diseases, including ulcers, atrophies, hyperkeratoses, cancers, granulomata, pigmentary and circulatory skin diseases and the somewhat more frequently seen so-called oil-acne and halogen-acne, toxic dermatitis and allergic contact-type eczematous dermatitis (= contact eczema) are encountered with overwhelming frequency. Thorough knowledge of these two diseases, therefore, is of utmost importance. Although at times, differential diagnosis between these two ailments seems nearly impossible, we personally feel obliged to discriminate between these two conditions as far as possible, because of the severe consequences which either of these diagnoses involve, especially in the field of occupational dermatology. Although both diseases can be clinically described as superficial inflammations of the skin which may show erythema, swelling, scaling, papules, vesicles, pustules, erosions, oozing etc., they differ in many respects, as will be seen from the following descriptions.

Dermatitis

Primary irritants induce toxic dermatitis in the majority of individuals on the very first contact, obviously due to their cytotoxic effect and not due to an acquired susceptibility of the patient. The reaction of irritation is relative, being influenced by the concentration, duration of exposure and local conditions. The resulting toxic dermatitis is usually fairly sharply delimited and restricted to the areas of direct contact with the noxa. The lesions may itch in the beginning, but later become stinging and painful. They may indeed display all the above mentioned phenomena, but usually the whole area shows a fairly uniform aspect, that is to say the whole plaque seems to be in the same stage of development. Thus, the whole area may be red and swollen; or red, swollen with vesicles rather evenly distributed over the whole site; or red, swollen and oozing over the whole surface; or brown red, less elevated and scaling. If an uneven distribution of symptoms is observed, this can often be correlated with maxima and minima of exposure or concentration; for instance, due to gravity the 'caudal' parts of the plaque may show a more severe or advanced picture if the noxa is a fluid. Histologically the noxious influence can be seen to spread from superficial to deeper layers of the skin, characterized by dyschromia, pyknosis, blisters (below str. corneum, filled predominantly with polymorphonuclear leucocytes) in the epithelium, and polynuclear infiltrate in the cutis. Discontinuation of the contact is generally followed by a rapid and steady process of (normal wound) healing in a couple of days up to 2 or 3 weeks. Renewed contact with the same noxa, but in a somewhat lower dosage (for instance 1/3 to 1/10 of the toxic dose) will generally be tolerated uneventfully. Thus after taking a few simple measures to lower skin-contact dose, the same work with the same noxa can be continued.

At the moment no supporting skin function test is available, unless one uses as such the negative outcome of patch tests in appropriate patch-testing concentrations with all contactants.

Contact eczema and other allergic manifestations

By contrast, in true *allergic sensitization*, only a minority of those exposed will acquire an allergic hypersensitivity unless one is dealing with an exceptionally potent sensitizer (*e.g.* one which is marked in the list of patch-test concentrations by Schwartz *et al.* 1957). Unless the noxa has combined toxic and sensitizing

References p. 39

potentialities, the first few or numerous contacts pass uneventfully. But suddenly, after the refractory period and the incubation period (see below) have elapsed without any symptoms, an allergic contact-type eczematous dermatitis may break out without any premonitory signs. This sequence of events must be extremely puzzling for laymen. Whereas previously the noxa has been well-tolerated for months or even years, thereafter even very small doses may initiate a recurrence of the contact eczema due to the hypersensitivity developed by the patient. Concerning the localization of the contact eczema, obviously more factors than simply the maximal exposure are influential: skin texture, the thickness of the skin, and if present previous (sub-clinical) toxic dermatitis play a more determining role concerning localization than in the case of toxic dermatitis. For instance, nail lacquer contact-eczema may to a lesser degree manifest itself in the nails and in the skin around the nails of the fingers where concentration and contact time are maximal, but it is mainly and most frequently localized on the eyelids, the sides of the neck and eventually on the ventral aspects of the elbows, due to scratching with the nails of these parts of the skin (which may have undergone a predisposing alteration due to local application of not fully skin-proof cosmetics).

Another striking feature of contact eczema of the hands is a tendency to involve the backs of the hands rather than the palms (at least during the initial acute phases) notwithstanding the fact that exposure of the palms is generally higher when working with solids or thick fluids.

Patches of eczema are nearly always fuzzily delimited from the surrounding normal skin and they tend to spread beyond the regions of direct contact with the noxious agent. A steady tendency to healing after discontinuation of contact, as seen in toxic dermatitis, is usually absent in contact eczema; on the contrary, an eczema tends to continue its exacerbating course in the first days after withdrawal of the noxious agent. In the beginning patches of contact eczema may show only redness

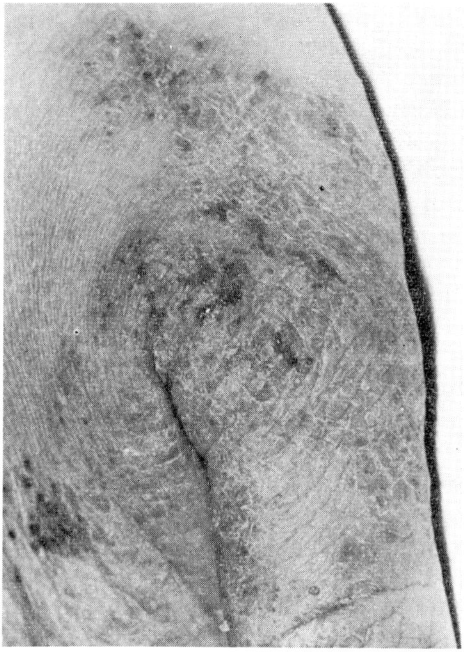

Fig. 2. Chronic contact eczema

with swelling, and this stage is easily confused with a beginning toxic dermatitis. But after a couple of days a remarkable polymorphism is seen: different parts of the patch show different stages of development: here scaling, there a cluster of vesicles, elsewhere a group of pinhead-sized erosions etc., and this pattern is continuously changing from time to time. These lesions itch and by scratching secondary infection may be introduced. In the final stages, pigmentation and lichenification may become manifest. Histologically the changes begin with a predominantly monocytic infiltrate high in the cutis (except in the very acute types of eczema in which polymorphonuclears may

References p. 39

be seen). These monocytic cells tend to spread upward. At the arrival of the monocytes in the lower layers of the epidermis, the basal membrane shows different staining qualities or disappears, the basal cells may balloon, areas of oedema collect inside and outside the lower prickle cells giving rise to spongiosis and finally to intraepidermal vesiculae, filled with lymphocytes rather than with polymorphonuclears, above which parakeratotic cornification is seen next to hyperkeratosis. The cells next to those involved stain as usual and do not show pyknosis. In chronic cases often marked acanthosis with elongation of the rete pegs may be seen, vesicle formation being absent.

In Europe, the skin disease just described is called contact eczema, in the Anglo-Saxon literature the name of allergic contact-type eczematous dermatitis has been coined by Sulzberger (1947). This author makes the following remarks in defending this nomenclature:

a. Allergic: the reaction is based on an acquired alteration in the capacity to react, which is highly specific, that is to say which is produced by previous exposure and manifested or elicited only on subsequent exposure to one and the same agent (or to an immunologic relative of that agent).

b. The disease is a result of a particular type of allergic reaction: it belongs to the category of delayed-type reactions. That is to say it is not characterized by an immediate response when the allergen (hapten) comes in contact with the sensitized tissues, but there is a latent period of several hours to several days before the clinical reaction becomes manifest. (For this reason patch-test readings after 24 and 48 hours and after some days, see p. 29.)

c. Contact-type dermatitis: the almost universal manner in which this disease is produced is by contact of the (sensitized) skin cells with the allergen (hapten) coming from without. There are exceptions to this rule, for instance: quinine dermatitis can be induced by ingestion or injection of quinine, etc. But the most usual manner of eliciting this response is through external contact. Therefore I call it "contact type". I do not use merely "contact" because the exceptions (quinine, etc.) belong to this group of diseases; that is the eczematous reactions in which the allergen (hapten) comes to the skin from within are still the same form and category of immunologic responses.

A few words can be added to the remarks of Sulzberger cited above, rather to enlarge the theoretical background than to point to really frequently occurring occupational allergic diseases.

From Rammazzini's days it has been known that flour can cause contact eczema as well as allergic asthma. Mayer observed both diseases due to *p*-phenylenediamine in the 1920's. Recently Key (1961) has summarized a number of substances from the industrial environment with the same potentialities: *inter alia* aliphatic polyamines, cobalt dust, complex platinum salts, formaldehyde, hexavalent chromium compounds, *p*-phenylenediamine, phthalic anhydride, toluene diisocyanates, wood dust. These substances thus can induce not only a contact-type allergy (delayed-type allergy) but also an immediate-type allergy sometimes occurring concomitantly. Realizing this last aspect, it is no wonder that the same author cites a number of substances which are known to be potential inducers of occupational urticaria; this is another form of immediate-type allergy, which, however, is a rare one. It is caused, among others, by complex platinum salts, aliphatic polyamines, ammonia, sulfur dioxide, formaldehyde, sodium sulfide.

Experimental and clinical details of contact eczema

In respect of the immunologic process of contact eczema, animal experiments made by a great many authors, among whom Haxthausen, and Frey and Wenk (1956, 1958) take a prominent place, are of utmost importance. Recent *communis opinio*, which can, for the greater part, be found in detail in Pillsbury *et al.* (1957), may be summarized as follows.

A simple chemical, acting as a hapten, applied to the surface

References p. 39

of the skin combines with some macromolecular substance (perhaps protein or mucopolysaccharide, which originate from the epithelium or stratum papillare cutis) to form a complete antigen within a limited lapse of time, say 24 hours. The complete antigen, presumably in phagocytized form, is transported through the lymphatics to the regional lymph nodes (which play an essential but not understood role) and from there it is carried through the blood stream to the reticuloendothelial system where it is stored. The complete antigen stimulates the R.E.S. cells to produce 'antibodies'. As nobody has ever isolated these 'antibodies' it may be better to speak of a certain transfer factor which is conferred on the lymphocytes of the blood stream, and

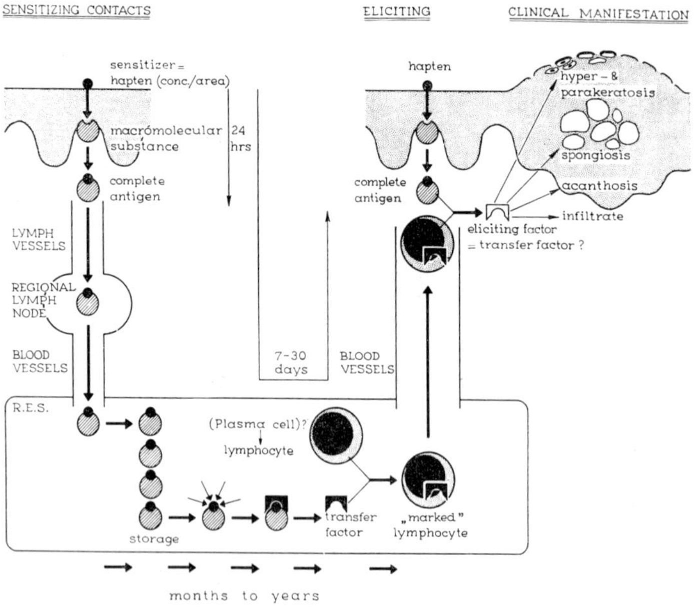

Fig. 3. Theory of allergic contact sensitization.

so hematogenously disseminated to the entire cutaneous system (one must bear in mind that circulating reagins, as seen in atopic states, are definitely not present in contact-allergic patients).

Thereafter the skin will show the reaction of contact eczema whenever there is surface contact with the sensitizer: after renewed penetration of the complete antigen to lymphocyte level in the skin, these lymphocytes presumably release the transfer factor, which conferred to sessile cells of the skin, starts the eczema reaction. This sequence of events (from the conjugation till the moment when a renewed contact may elicit a contact-eczema reaction for the first time) takes at least seven days with potent sensitizers but may take up to 30 days or more with weaker ones. The R.E.S. remains active in conferring the peculiar transfer factor to lymphocytes for months or even years in the absence of any stimulating factor from outside. During this period every renewed contact of the sensitizer with the skin will be followed (within a couple of hours, 6–24 or more) by an outbreak of the clinical manifestations of contact eczema. A couple of weeks after complete obliteration of the sensitizer from the skin, this may appear clinically healed, but in a pathological sense the patient remains affected for months or years until at last a new contact with the sensitizer eventually proves that he has lost his peculiar capacity to react (new refractory period).

One can discern a number of periods in the evolution of contact eczema, *viz.:* the refractory period, the incubation period, the period of clinical manifestations and the period of clinical cure. These periods are schematically drawn in Fig. 4 from which, moreover, it can be seen in which periods preventive measures or replacement management may be effective and during which periods a positive patch test may be encountered. As may be observed from the picture, the patch test sometimes gives a negative result in the very early days of a very acute and extensive contact eczema ('positive anergy').

Moreover, it can be seen that it takes 3 or 4 weeks after dis-

References p. 39

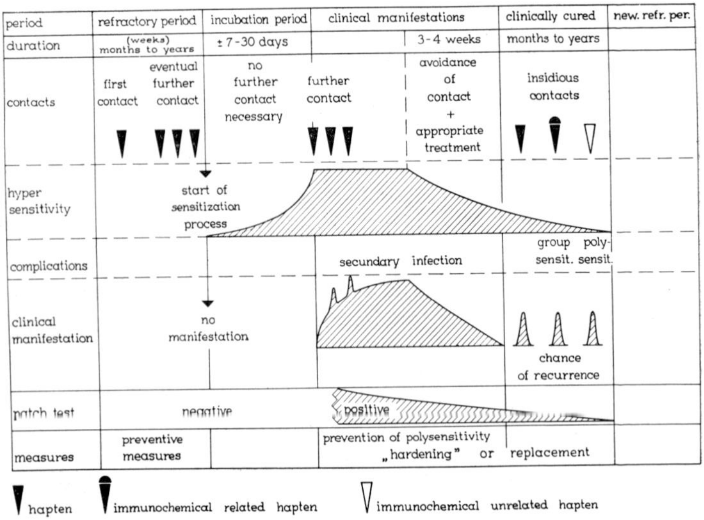

Fig. 4. Scheme of contact hypersensitivity.

continuation of contact with the sensitizer before the skin will be clinically healed again. This is the time necessary for a complete renewal of the epithelium. Such healed-skin sites seem perfectly normal, but especially in the first weeks after clinical healing they remain vulnerable physiologically. The hyper-irritability is manifest not only specifically when sub-reactive concentrations of the particular antigen are applied but also non-specifically: irritants incapable of affecting normal skin may produce reaction in such healed areas.

For several reasons, steady healing may be delayed:

a. Discontinuation of work-contact with the sensitizer may seem complete, but contact may continue unknowingly: a sensitized quinine-worker must stop drinking tonics; a tetramethyl-thiuram disulfide-sensitized worker must stop using a special brand of soap or special mark of rubber gloves, he must not eat certain kinds of food and it may be better to avoid treatment with antabuse for alcohol addiction (possible group sensitization).

b. Sensitization may appear not to be so strikingly specific as might be expected theoretically. Thus chemically related substances may act as elicitors of the reaction: group specificity. The condition then may persist because of secondary allergens which the patient is unknowingly absorbing or contacting. A *p*-phenylenediamine-sensitized worker may react on contact with azo dyes, picric acid or sulfa therapeutics, etc. (Mayer 1954). A hydrazine hydrochloride-sensitized worker may react to isoniazid therapy for tuberculosis (Fost *et al.* 1959). This phenomenon of group specificity must be borne in mind in questions related to replacement and therapy.

c. As dermatitic skin, whatever the origin of inflammation, is more readily sensitized than normal skin, it may happen that more than one substance appears to have acted as sensitizer: poly(valent)sensitization. Thus in patients sensitized for ethoxylin resins a concomitant sensitization for the aliphatic polyamines, used in curing these resins, may rather be often encountered (Malten 1956, see p. 133). For this reason it is also of the utmost importance to use bland local therapeutics especially in the acute phases of contact eczema (no locally applied antibiotics (Kooy 1961) or mercury-containing ointments). In this respect it may therefore be wise to apply dressings to acute eczemata in order to eliminate immediately all untoward exogenous influences.

'HARDENING' (ACQUIRED TOLERANCE)

From the foregoing it may be clear that withdrawal from (work-)contact with the sensitizer is the classical method of solving the contact-eczema problem. Peck *et al.* (1945) have pointed to a second way of handling patients with industrial contact eczema, which may be used by experts in this field: that is 'hardening' the patient against the industrial sensitizer he is exposed to. By 'hardening' is meant the disappearance or the failure of reappearance of an allergic contact-type dermatitis in sensitized individuals on continued or repeated exposure in industry to the sensitizing chemical. The interested reader should peruse the cited article in the original.

Malten (1958) observed hardening in sensitizations to azo dyes, phenolformaldehyde-type resins and chromate. That hardening seems to occur spontaneously in quite a number of industrially exposed workers must be concluded from re-evaluation of large groups. These individuals show, or have shown, minor ailments with a tendency to heal spontaneously, notwithstanding continuation of industrial contact below a certain critical level. With patch testing, they present medium to strong positive reactions to substances with which they are in continuous contact during their work. Under expert control, hardening may be tried, but in our opinion only by volunteers. Success depends upon the initial level of sensitivity and the nature of the allergen involved. The hardening phenomenon is temporary: after absence from his job for a period of time the worker (and the physician) may be distressed to discover that he again reacts upon re-exposure.

PATCH-TESTING PROCEDURE AND INTERPRETATION

In expert hands, the patch test is of utmost importance in identifying the substance or substances to which the patient is hypersensitive. The substance to be tested is placed on a square piece of cotton measuring *ca.* 7 × 7 mm and is then applied to the skin of the back, presuming that no clinical symptoms have recently appeared at that site. The piece of cotton is covered with a square piece of cellophane measuring *ca.* 17 × 17 mm, fastened by adhesive tape measuring *ca.* 50 × 60 mm. The patch remains *in situ* for at least 24 hours, when it is carefully removed. The degree of reaction is read 10 to 15 minutes after removal of the patch in order to let eventual adhesive-tape reactions

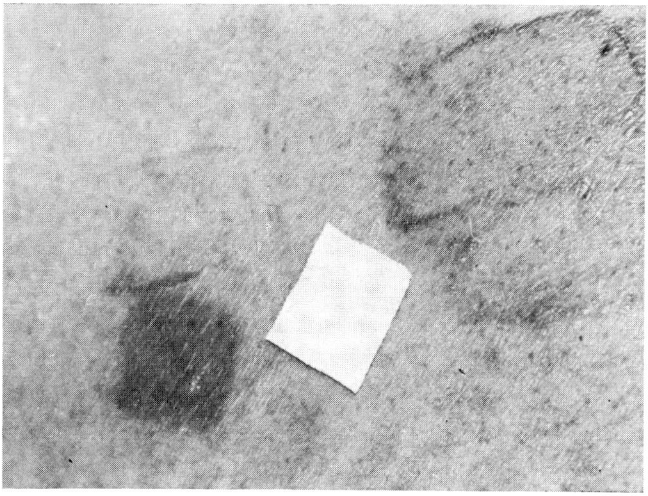

Fig. 5. Patch-testing results. Left: toxic reaction (primary irritation). Middle: patch size. Right: allergic reaction (sensitizer).

subside. The reaction is read again 48 hours after application (at which time reading is often augmented in comparison with the 24-hour reading) and at intervals of 3 to 5 days in order to record late reactions (which may be due to one of three reasons: *viz.* low concentration, low sensitivity, inherent slow reaction to exposure).

As the purpose of the test is to evaluate hypersensitivity, the concentration of the substance under investigation and the vehicle in which it is dissolved should be chosen in such a way as to be non-irritant to normally sensitive persons. If the substance is not named in lists for patch-testing concentrations published by Schwartz *et al.* (1957), Nater (1961), Van Vloten (1950), Key *et al.* (1961), Schultheiss (1959), Malten (1956, 1958), the physician must himself estimate an appropriate testing concentration and vehicle. This is always true when mixtures of unknown concentrations, composition and grade of impurity, which are often encountered in industries, must be handled.

References p. 39

(This is the chief reason why various authors recommend different testing concentrations.) Moreover the choice of the vehicle (which in itself must of course be non-toxic) may be of great influence: a given concentration of the substance in one vehicle may be toxic, in another harmless.

The first thing to do, if working with substances of unknown composition, is to find out the toxic concentration, which may be defined as the concentration in a given vehicle which causes toxic reaction of any grade in half the number of the normal volunteers tested (probit-analysis) under patch-testing conditions, after 24 hours. To minimize the number and the severity of effects in the group of volunteers, the investigator himself may be the first 'experimental animal' because he will remove the patch as soon as a reaction appears and knows best how to remove the substance under investigation from his skin.

Strangely, nobody knows how large a safety margin must be allowed below the toxic concentration in order to avoid:

a. Testing with a concentration which is still too high for one or several individuals in a large group of normally sensitive persons, as a result of which a positive reaction of irritation may be misinterpreted as sensitization in a patient already sensitized by some other factor, whose clinically sound skin areas may, moreover, show greater irritability than those of normal individuals (*e.g.*, 1% $K_2Cr_2O_7$ in aqua: 'false positive reaction').

b. Using a concentration which may be too low to reveal low-grade sensitization (*e.g.*, 0.001% $K_2Cr_2O_7$ in aqua: 'false negative reaction').

Here, science ends and art begins: it is our impression that working with 1/3 to 1/5 of the toxic concentration (depending on the slope of the probit-analysis curve) may be safe, provided the investigator is alert to the type of reaction read on the patients back. Apart from a number of misleading positive reactions which are known to occur (pustulae after contact with copper and nickel salts, petechiae after cobalt salts, miliaria rubra due to moist microclimate), one must distinguish a positive toxic reaction from a positive allergic reaction; this may be difficult especially in low-grade reactions, but not hopeless if one bears in mind the following points:

1. A primary toxic reaction shows the clinical picture of toxic dermatitis with the most intense signs in the caudal part; it has about the size and shape of the applied square piece of cotton and is sharply delimited. After removal of the patch, which lowers the testing concentration, healing begins at once.

2. The reaction of sensitization shows one or another stage of contact eczema, which spreads in a rounded plaque beyond the scope of the square piece of cotton, with fuzzy borders. Twenty-four hours after removing the patch the reaction may be even more severe notwithstanding lowering of contact concentration. The pinpoint-sized vesiculae are best seen with tangential illumination from a pocket lighter.

If one is nevertheless not sure of the character of the reaction the testing procedure should be repeated (preferably not around the ninth day after the first patch test) with a slightly lower concentration (say 80%). In that case a toxic reaction may not appear, whereas a contact eczema reaction may still develop. For further details the reader is referred to Pillsbury *et al.* (1957).

We want to make a final remark: Patch testing in the acute stages of the contact eczema should be avoided for several reasons: First the possible non-specific irritability of the patient's whole skin including seemingly normal areas. Second the possibility of focal reaction which must be feared especially in the acute phases, but which may occur in the chronic period as well if the test concentration is rather high, the contact time rather long or the patient highly sensitive. Applying the sensitizer to the skin in a patch test under such circumstances may give a recrudescence of the original contact eczema lesions. Third, because in the acute initial stages of the contact eczema the patient may show a so-called positive anergy for the sensitizer (negative patch test). A clear-cut positive reaction may be elicited when tested one or two weeks later.

References p. 39

A list of patch-testing concentrations of several substances connected with plastics is given on p. 237.

DIFFERENTIAL DIAGNOSIS

In differential diagnosis one must think of eczema mycoticum, eczema seborrhoicum, eczema nummulare and two entities which deserve special interest *viz.*: *a.* desiccation dermatitis (= housewives' dermatitis), and *b.* dyshidrosis, because both may originate from working conditions.

ad a. The barrier-zone of Szakall (= stratum conjunctum of the horny layer) and the stratum granulosum contain hygroscopic substances which, with help of the surface water in oil emulsion (in winter), try to maintain 10% moisture in the stratum corneum, which is of utmost importance for the integrity of the barrier-zone. In people who easily develop chapping skin, a certain deficiency of hygroscopic substances and of oil (to hold water) may be supposed. On the other hand, intensive washing out of these substances by frequent contact with 'soap' and water, or solvents, may also lower the water content of the stratum, with rupturing of the barrier-zone as a consequence. Whereas an intact barrier-zone prevents water and ions from penetrating into the prickle-cell layer, this route is now open. This may result in a low-grade inflammation of the superficial layers of the skin, even histologically resembling contact eczema: spotty (due to the breaks in the barrier?) spongiosis, para- and hyper-keratosis, lymphocytic perivascular infiltrate in the cutis. The clinical picture shows rather sharply demarcated patches of bright, but not intensive redness with scaling: *i.e.* toxic dermatitis. Therapy consists in bathing in 0.9% NaCl solution and thereafter applying a water-holding cream or ointment.

ad b. Dyshidrosis is characterized by multiple, rather deep-seated clear, pinpoint- to pinhead-sized vesicles, exclusively on the volar aspects of the hands and the sides of the fingers. In over 30% this reaction can be seen as an allergic reaction complicating tinea pedis. If this condition is not present on the feet, dyshidrosis may be associated with focal infections of cocci, fungi or yeasts elsewhere in the body. The condition may be observed during exacerbations of atopic dermatitis and in some cases one can find arguments to regard it as a true contact eczema. Finally, some authors think of real occlusion of sweat gland pores. In a number of these patients Mali *et al.* (1961) have succeeded in finding by direct intracutaneous prick tests, corroborated by positive passive anaphylaxis tests, symptoms pointing to circulating antibodies. The condition of these patients was exacerbated after inhalation of the incriminated antigens, such as potassium bichromate, cinnamyl aldehyde, benzoic acid, *o*-cresol, turpentine and flour. In 4 out of 7 patients described, the patch-test reaction remained negative. It goes without saying that evaluation of the volatile sensitizers which act through inhalation in these cases is extremely difficult. Finding the noxious agent in these cases depends mostly on the intelligence of the patient himself and often takes more than one year of close observation. In this respect the well-informed industrial medical officer may be in a more advantageous position, because all particulars of the working conditions are known to him.

SOME REMARKS ABOUT TREATMENT

In the treatment of toxic dermatitis in the acute oozing stages application of soothing wet dressings (*e.g.* Dalibour water* without tinctura croci), bland emulsions or, in the less-acute stages, of water-containing creams (*e.g.* Emulgide 10%, ol. arachidis 10%, methylparabene 0.5%, aqua ad 100) may suffice. In the treatment of contact eczema it is of the utmost importance to prevent development of polyvalent sensitization. That means, it is imperative to dress the skin lesions (be it with a thin and non-

* Eau Dalibour: R Cupri sulfatis 1; zinci sulfatis 3.5, aquae camforatae ad 100; 2–3 tablespoons per litre water.

References p. 39

occlusive dressing) and to use bland, non-sensitizing therapeutic agents. Moreover, the physical properties of the local therapeutics are of greater importance than the chemical ones. Usually the Dalibour-water phase of treatment needs only be very short (or can be omitted). One may continue with pasta zinci oleosa (zinc oxide 60, ol. olivarum ad 100) to which a small percentage of sulfur praecipitatis or vioform can be added to impede 'secondary infection'. In the later stages, if this paste should cause too strong drying, 20 to 50% lanoline may be added, and the content of specific therapeutics (sulfur, vioform, tar) may be augmented. Local corticosteroids (and *a fortiori* systemic administration) are useless before the contact with the sensitizer has been stopped, and in our opinion, are seldom helpful thereafter. In fact they may mask the clinical course and thus may obviate disclosure of important contributing factors in the pathogenesis of the sensitization. Moreover, the ointment base in which topical corticosteroids are offered by pharmaceutical industries is generally unknown and often inappropriate for the stage in which the contact eczema abides.

Local application of sulfonamides or antibiotics is a mistake; they are seldom necessary (and can be replaced in these instances by sulfur and vioform), they may sensitize in a far greater number of cases and are a source of resistant cocci.

Desensitizing treatment is generally unsuccessful in contact eczema.

REFERENCES

FOST, J. and N. HJÖRTH, Contact dermatitis from hydrazine hydrochloride in soldering flux; cross sensitization to apresoline and isoniazid. *Acta Dermato-Venereol.*, 39 (1959) 82.

FREY, J. R. and P. WENK, Experimentelle Untersuchungen zur Pathogenese des Kontaktekzems. *Dermatologica*, 112 (1956) 265.

FREY, J. R. and P. WENK, Über die Funktion der regionalen Lymphknoten bei der Entstehung des Dinitrochlorbenzol-Kontaktekzems am Meerschweinchen. *Dermatologica*, 116 (1958) 243.

KEY, M. M., Some unusual allergic reactions in industry. *Arch. Dermatol.*, 83 (1961) 3.

KEY, M. M., V. B. PERONE and D. J. BIRMINGHAM, Patch testing in dermatitis from the newer resins. *J. Occupational Med.*, 3 (1961) 361.

KOOY, R., Allergic contact dermatitis due to Neomycin. *S. African Med. J.*, 35 (1961) 406.

LANE, C., Industrial dermatoses. *J. Am. Med. Assoc.*, 118 (1942) 613.

MALI, J. W. H., K. E. MALTEN and F. C. J. VAN NEER, Eczeem van de handen. *Geneesk. Bl.*, 50 (1961) 1.

MALTEN, K. E., *Beroepsekzeem bij het verwerken van kunststoffen*, Thesis, Amsterdam, 1956.

MALTEN, K. E., Occupational eczema in those who print cotton by hand. In *Occupational Allergy*, Stenfert Kroese, Leiden, 1958.

MAYER, R. L., Group sensitization to compounds of quinone structure. *Progress in Allergy*, Vol. IV. Karger, Basel, 1954.

NATER, J. P., *Chromaateczeem*, Thesis, Amsterdam, 1961.

PECK, S. M., J. G. GANT and L. SCHWARTZ, 'Hardening' in industrial allergic dermatitis. *Ind. Med.*, 14 (1945) 214.

PILLSBURY, D. M., W. B. SHELLEY and A. M. KLIGMAN, *Dermatology*, Saunders, Philadelphia, 1957.

SCHULTHEISS, E., *Gummi und Ekzem*, Cantor, Aulendorf, 1959.

SCHWARTZ, L., L. TULIPAN and D. J. BIRMINGHAM, *Occupational Diseases of the Skin*, Lea & Febiger, Philadelphia, 1957.

SULZBERGER, M., Contact-type eczematous dermatitis. *J. Allergy*, 18 (1947) 176.

VLOTEN, TH. J. VAN, *Een onderzoek bij allergische huidverschijnselen veroorzaakt door sulfa-preparaten*, Thesis, Amsterdam, 1950.

5

Phenoplasts and aminoplasts

PHYSICO-CHEMICAL PROPERTIES, APPLICATION

Phenoplasts and aminoplasts are polycondensation resins; it is possible to stop the condensation-equilibrium reaction at any desired moment (see p. 8).

Semi-cured intermediates may be formed and, as such, transported and processed further. The final curing is achieved by means of temperature, pressure or curing agents; this often takes place in open systems.

Since both groups of resins have somewhat similar hygienic aspects, they are discussed together in one chapter.

Phenoplasts

These resins are polycondensates of *phenols* (phenol, cresol, xylenol, resorcinol, *p*-alkylphenols) and *aldehydes* (formaldehyde, acroleïn, furfural, benzaldehyde, ketones). In the majority of cases *phenol* and *formaldehyde* (as formalin: 20–40 % in water) are used: the *o*- and *p*-places in the phenol molecule are cross-linked by means of CH_2-bridges derived from the formaldehyde (see p. 9).

Two types of polycondensation may be distinguished:

Acid condensation: phenols react as bifunctional compounds and semi-cured, linear, low-molecular intermediates (Novolak) occur, cured in the application phase by adding hexamethylenetetramine (= 'hexa'), which at high temperatures produces formaldehyde and ammonia (alkaline condensation).

Alkaline condensation: the phenols react as tri-functional compounds: tri-dimensional net structures result (thermosetting under pressure). The condensation reaction may be stopped at different stages: A-resin (Resol), a liquid and soluble low condensate; B-resin (Resitol), still soluble but with elastic properties; C-resin (Resit), completely cured, solid and insoluble. It is possible to mix the Resol resin with fillers and pigments, and thereupon to cure the mixture into a Resitol by heating. The semi-cured resin is pressed into moulding compounds (tablets or powder), which are still biologically active. According to Archangelskaja (1957) moulding powder still contained even 7.2% free phenol and 9.1% free formaldehyde. The final curing into thermosetting Resit stage takes place generally in heated moulding presses. Lacquers or glues may be cured by adding acid without heating (acid cold-curing).

It should be noted that substituted stilbene compounds may be formed as intermediates (endocrinological effects have not been reported).

The phenoplasts find many applications:
- lacquer, either as 100% resin or as a modified resin (*e.g.*, with colophonium). As phenol compounds, *p*-alkylphenols are often used;
- casting resin (alkaline condensation);
- moulding compound (with or without filler);
- glue, *e.g.* for metals or leather;
- impregnation for paper and wood, yielding 'hard board', etc.

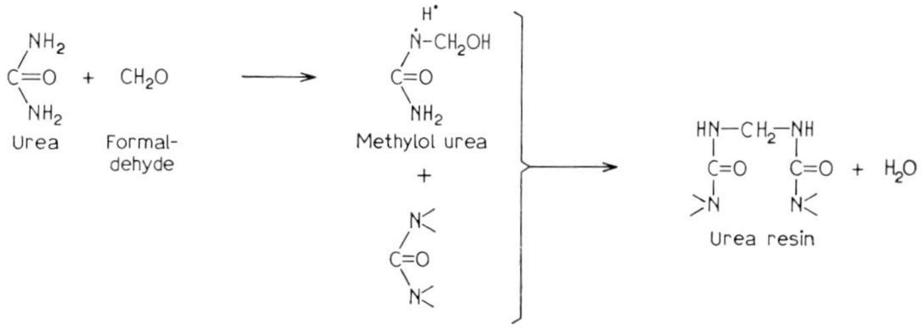

References p. 54

Aminoplasts (Carbamid resins)

Well-known resins in this group are:

– *urea resins*, thermosetting plastics, produced from urea and formaldehyde.

During acid-curing biologically active formaldehyde may be set free (ether-links are converted into CH_2-links). This reaction proceeds as follows:

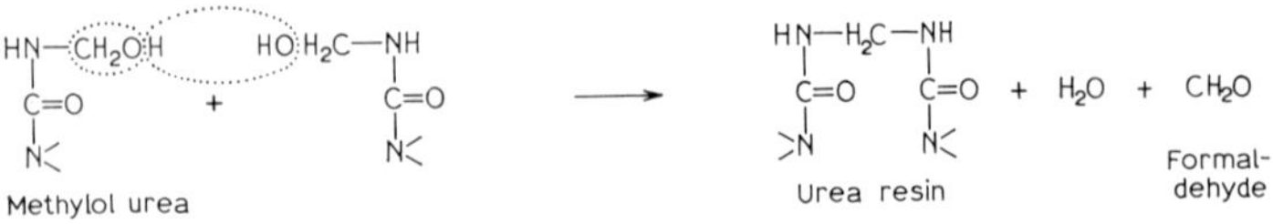

In the urea-formaldehyde resin, hexamethylenetetramine acts as a *stabilizer* to prevent the resin from hardening before it is moulded; less than 1 % of it is used in the resin (Schwarz *et al.* 1957).

– *melamine resins*, from melamine (= 2,4,6-triamino-1,3,5-triazine) and formaldehyde.

– *thiourea resins*, from thiourea and formaldehyde.

The aminoplasts are applied, among others, as lacquer (hot-curing enamel), moulding compounds, glue, textile finish ('non-iron'), foam plastic.

Decomposition

Decomposition of phenoplasts and aminoplasts may occur by heating. According to Bolton *et al.* (1942) phenoplasts produce CO and H_2 above 540 °. Sendroy *et al.* (1952) sampled the gases and vapours emanating from a phenoplast-coating of a sub-marine engine running for a period of 96 hours at 150, 200, 250 and 300 °. Only the CO level rose to toxic concentrations for rats; CO_2, NH_3, phenol and formaldehyde did not reach these levels. Berger *et al.* (1947) mentioned the occurrence of cyanogen (–CN) compounds, although in low concentrations. According to Schaefer (1953) even aromatic hydrocarbons (amongst others benzene) could be produced by decomposition of phenoplasts. Melamine resins may disintegrate into CO, HCN and NH_3; the presence of fillers increased the CO concentration (Berger *et al.* 1947). Elkins (1959) and Coleman (1959) emphasized the greater hazard from CO in contrast to HCN in burning N-containing plastics. However, the experimental data of Moss *et al.* (1951) should be borne in mind: pyrolysis of melamine yielded HCN and pyrolysis of melamine resins in addition CO; simultaneous exposure to low concentrations of CO and HCN indicated a synergistic effect in rats: the excitation and hyperpnoea (result of HCN) increased the CO uptake.

INDUSTRIAL TOXICOLOGY

The data regarding the components may be shortly reviewed. The toxicology of the *phenols* has been described extensively by Von Oettingen (1949).

Phenol is corrosive for skin and mucosa. The noxa is absorbed through the skin. The acute toxic effect for oral uptake is similar to that of percutaneous absorption: asthenia, headache, vertigo, tinnitus, irregular respiration, circulatory failure, coma, death. Oral or percutaneous uptake of 1 g may be fatal. Chronic intoxication is seen very seldom: symptoms arising from the gastrointestinal tract and central nervous system, damage to liver and kidney. Because of the low volatility (vapour pressure 1 mm Hg at 44.8 °) the industrial hazard in respect of inhalation is very small, in contrast to the possibility of percutancous absorption.

Formaldehyde, a volatile gas, is irritating to the mucosae of eyes and air passages. The following effects may occur: bronchitis, dermatitis, rhinitis, oropharyngitis, conjunctivitis. The irritation proves to be a good warning signal: serious acute intoxication (pulmonary oedema, coma) rarely occurs. However a habituation to irritating levels may be quickly established. The toxicology of *aldehydes* has been extensively covered by U.S. Public Health Service (1945) and Henson (1959): the toxicity of

References p. 54

the lower aldehydes decreases with chain length; unsaturated aldehydes are more toxic than those saturated. *Urea* is non-toxic; as to *melamine*, no adequate data are reported.

Industrial toxicological effects from the *production* of phenoplasts were recognized in the first years of the introduction of synthetic plastics. Weger (1927) and Baader (1932) referred to headache, asthenia, disturbance of peripheral nervous sensitivity, irregular ventilation, retrosternal oppression, tachycardia, eye irritation under bad ventilation conditions. Harris (1953) examined 25 workers who for at least 5 years had made urea resins. For the greater part of the time the formaldehyde concentration was below 10 p.p.m., maximal 30 p.p.m. Minor reversible dermatosis had occurred in 4, mostly reversible lymphocytosis in 6, and 4 workers complained of slight dyspnoea (amongst them one hypertensive state, one asthma). A case of occupational allergic asthma in a urea-formaldehyde worker developed after accidental excessive inhalation of a mixture of formaldehyde–butanol–turpentine. Tara (1956) who described this case, however, emphasized the relative rarity of allergic respiratory disease in workers in these factories. This was confirmed by Zielhuis (1960), who examined 37 workers employed for 2 years at least in a factory producing pheno- and aminoplasts and alkyd resins. Apart from 9 dermatoses in the occupational history, no chronic bronchitic manifestations were observed; laboratory analysis did not reveal any disturbance of liver function or hematopoiesis.

Since the second world war the '*shell-moulding process*' (Form-Masken Verfahren of Croning) has been introduced in the *foundries:* pheno- and aminoplasts are used as binder for moulding sand. Quooss (1959), Banik (1959) and Tübich *et al.* (1960) described the hygienic complications. Principal steps in the shell-moulding process are: preforming metal patterns, coating of sand with a thermosetting resin, investing or blowing resin–sand mixture on to heated pattern, curing shell mould in oven and assembling the two mould halves by means of adhesive thermosetting resin. A shell mould of 0.5–1 cm thickness is formed. As moulding material most frequently a mixture of fine silica (sometimes Zr, olivine, Al, Mg, chromite), 3–6% resin (mostly phenoplast) and hexamethylenetetramine is used: during mixing, exposure to these compounds may occur. In the oven the curing process causes the emanation of NH_3, aldehydes and phenols, which may cause a highly irritant atmosphere. Particularly during pouring and shake-out significant quantities of CO are released. The solvents used for the resin, for the parting compounds (silicone or wax) and for cleaning of the moulds constitute a real problem: alcohols (*e.g.* methanol), chlorinated (*e.g.* carbon tetrachloride), aliphatic and aromatic (*e.g.* benzene) hydrocarbons. If urea resin is applied, phosphoric acid is used as a hardener (dermatitis, eye irritation). Hygienic complications arise particularly from exposure to silica, CO, solvents, odorous and irritating agents; skin diseases (formaldehyde, hexa) may be present in up to 15–20% of the moulders and mixing operators. Banik (1959) drew attention to the strong odour pervading the whole department and attaching itself to the clothes of the workers. He advised installing two dressing rooms, one for doffing the dirty working clothes and the other for donning street-clothes, separated by a washing-room. Another serious problem is the odorous emanation into the air in the vicinity of the mill.

In the *textile industry* urea and melamine resins are used as finish in order to make the clothes crease-resistant. Several authors have mentioned hygienic complications. Quooss (1959) examined 53 textile workers, exposed to formaldehyde (below 18 p.p.m.) and pyridine. He observed several dermatoses (formaldehyde allergy), gastric disorders (presumably by pyridine), bronchitic symptoms and eosinophilia, lymphocytosis and toxic granulations in the peripheral blood. Ettinger *et al.* (1955) and Giel *et al.* (1956) mentioned conjunctivitis (by formaldehyde vapour), keratitis (by flakes of uncured resin) and contact dermatitis in sewing women. They recommended the following

References p. 54

preventive measures: extra ventilation, curing in acid medium, washing the clothes in soda, personal protective devices. Tara (1956) even observed a case of asthmatic dyspnoea in a clothing store: dyspnoea occurred at first during ironing, but later on even at the slightest contact. Also Bourne *et al.* (1959) and Le Coulant *et al.* (1961) mentioned similar symptoms in personnel and customers of textile shops.

In the *paper industry*, the application of pheno- and aminoplasts has also been a cause of occupational disability. Bompart *et al.* (1959) examined workers in an abrasive paper industry. Textile or paper is impregnated with phenoplasts in an alcoholic solution, sprayed with a scouring powder, and afterwards cured and cut. During the winter particularly, complaints were received concerning irritation of the eyes and gastric disturbances. Probably as a result of idiosyncrasy and of relatively high exposure, 4 cases of asthma occurred. Several cases of dermatosis were seen, probably conditioned also by detergents, antihistaminic ointments and mechanical irritation. Processing by hand yielded one or more symptoms in 20 out of 26 workers, mechanical processing, however, only in 10 out of 35 workers. Morrill (1961) observed symptoms of itching eyes, sore throat, sleep disturbances, thirst in the morning in workers engaged in a paper-conditioning process; urea resin was applied to paper in order to prevent shrinkage. Increased ventilation improved the working conditions. Quooss (1959) noted the nauseating odour occurring from sawing the so-called 'hard paper', 'hard tissue' (with phenoplasts impregnated and laminated papers and tissues), particularly if the saws became blunt, causing the temperature to rise.

Urea resins may be used for insulating *foam plastics*. Amongst German railway crews, Baader *et al.* (1957) observed eye irritation and asthmatic dyspnoea during installation of foam packets in cold-storage wagons. In a crew of 25 workers, 16 complained of irritation of the air passages, 2 of burning pain in the eyes, 8 of anorexia and sickness. Upon physical examination eosinophilia was observed in 5 of the crew, bronchitis in 12, emphysema in 5, and chronic conjunctivitis in 4. The cause of all these troubles was presumably formaldehyde.

Pheno- and aminoplasts may also be used in *glueing systems, e.g.* shoe glue and Redux glue: after preparation with chlorinated hydrocarbons and chromic acid. Aluminium metal surfaces are coated with Redux liquid (alcoholic solution of semi-cured phenoplasts), sprayed with Redux powder (polyvinyl formaldehyde), and glued together under pressure at 150°. Sporadic cases of contact eczema due to Redux liquid were observed by Malten (1956); asthmatic dyspnoea due to glues has also been reported in three workers (Tara 1956).

The processing of *moulding compounds* (powder or tablets) may also give rise to serious troubles. A case of bronchiolitis obliterans has been described, presumably due to inhalation of phenoplasts (Ludwig 1935). Archangelskaja (1957) observed headache, irritability, asthenia, anorexia, dry coughing, hoarseness, thoracic pains amongst workers handling moulding compounds; dermatoses occurred particularly during the first months of exposure, the other symptoms increased in intensity with continuing exposure. Hanslian *et al.* (1958) even described ulcers and necroses of the nasal mucosa in workers handling urea-formaldehyde moulding compounds.

The acid curing (by HCl) of *paints* with a urea-formaldehyde basis under bad ventilation conditions caused a severe and long-lasting asthmatic attack, probably due to the emanating formaldehyde (Zielhuis 1961).

INDUSTRIAL DERMATOLOGY

Phenol and *formaldehyde* are both primary irritants and sensitizers. Phenol sensitization occurs less frequently than formaldehyde sensitization, presumably partly due to the volatility of the latter. No untoward effects from *urea* are known. *Hexamethylenetetramine* decomposes by heating into formaldehyde

References p. 54

and ammonia, the latter being an irritant and both are possible causes of allergic urticaria (Key 1961). *Melamine* is not mentioned in literature, but *methylol-melamine* may sensitize (Malten 1962b).

Lockey (1944) gave an excellent description of the processing hazards of phenol-formaldehyde and urea-formaldehyde resins. Hypersensitivity to hexamethylenetetramine and formaldehyde was the main cause of occupational dermatitis. Hypersensitivity to phenol was found in a lesser degree. Apparently urea hypersensitivity was not observed. Allergic contact dermatitis may occur in users of moulded phenol-formaldehyde and urea-formaldehyde resin wares if not all the 'hexa' is combined; the same may be true of phenol. Wilde (1959) described 4 cases of contact hypersensitivity to the rims of spectacles made of an undefined plastic. The lesions promptly healed after change to another brand of spectacles. All showed positive patch tests to formaldehyde.

Lefaux (1954) reported on moulding phenoplasts at a temperature of 200° and a pressure of 200 to 300 kg/cm^2. He observed contact sensitization predominantly amongst men working in the vicinity of the presses due to evaporation of the components phenol, formaldehyde and ammonia. The fully cured-out condensates are, in his opinion, inert, but in cases in which not fully cured resins are used, that is to say in cases where phenoplasts or aminoplasts in solution or suspension are used as adhesives, (textile) finish or lacquers, sensitizations may occur due to excess of unreacted reactants (phenol, amines, formaldehyde). Schwartz *et al.* (1943) reported contact allergic dermatitis from resin glue in war industries. Among others they mentioned the use of *hydrazines* as catalysts (hydrazine compounds have been reported to cause contact sensitization in recent years by Fost *et al.* (1959), Schultheiss (1959) and Malten (1962a). In a number of cases hydrazine-sensitized people showed a group specificity to therapeutics such as apresoline and isoniazid which may have serious implications). Schwartz *et al.* showed that these resins also had primary skin-irritant properties. The risk of manual contact with glues has also been stressed by Brunner (1962), who saw 6 cases of sensitivity to formaldehyde.

Bourret *et al.* (1958) published a paper on industrial dermatoses due to formaldehyde and its industrial derivatives: phenoplasts and aminoplasts. The type and the appearance of clinical manifestations corresponded to a high degree with the concentration of formaldehyde in the solutions under observation. In 9 cases they performed patch tests, and in all 9 formaldehyde was the only substance found to have acted as the sensitizer. The refractory period was rather short: a few days or weeks; females especially between 40 and 60 years of age were easily sensitized. Glass (1961) reported an outbreak of formaldehyde dermatitis in a factory manufacturing phenol, melamine and urea resins. In addition to manual contact, the workers were exposed to 16–30 p.p.m. formaldehyde. Preventive measures controlled this outbreak effectively; the concentration in air dropped to 2–5 p.p.m.

Malten (1958) investigated the cases of ten cobblers who contracted a contact eczema of the hands, wrists and sometimes of the face due to a new additive to a classical latex adhesive. This additive was a polycondensate made from *p-tert.*-butylphenol and formaldehyde. All ten cobblers showed a positive patch-test reaction to the added polycondensate as well as to the *p-tert.*-butylphenol component; two showed a positive reaction to phenol (group specificity?); a positive patch test to formaldehyde was seen only twice. These formaldehyde hypersensitivities might be explained as being due to contact with residues of antimycotic powders in the shoes repaired. A number of shoe glues with different fancy names also appeared to give positive patch-test reactions, apparently because these glues contained the same additive. Thus, in most cases a change to a differently labelled glue did not result in amelioration and some of the cobblers had already concluded that the shoe adhesive could not be the cause of their contact eczema. It is obviously necessary to

References p. 54

indicate on the bottle the components of a mixture that are to come into intimate contact with the skin during application or use.

Schwartz (1941) found cases of contact eczema caused by handling fabrics on which urea-formaldehyde finish was used in amounts of 8–100 mg of formaldehyde per 100 g yarn, and showed this to be the cause of the contact eczemas. Bourne *et al.* (1959) found the same range of formaldehyde concentrations in melamine- and urea-formaldehyde-treated rayon. In several dress shops the air contained from 0.13 to 0.45 p.p.m. of formaldehyde. According to Le Coulant *et al.* (1961) a percentage of 0.2% free formaldehyde in the finish is generally accepted. Methods for determination of the formaldehyde content of textiles were given by Roff (1956) and Blohm (1959).

However, Gaul *et al.* (1949) patch-tested a formaldehyde-sensitive patient with a polycondensate of *o*-methylolphenol (known sensitizer, occurring in textile finish, made from phenol and formaldehyde) and they obtained negative results. Thus in this polycondensation-product formaldehyde is present in only subliminal concentrations.

The same may be concluded from recent investigations made by Malten (1962b, 1963) who patch-tested 28 patients who anamnesically and clinically suffered from a textile-finish contact eczema. Only 7 showed positive patch tests to formaldehyde, which always were combined with positive patch-test reactions with a number of compounds made by the reaction of formaldehyde with other reactants, for instance: dimethylolurea (12/28 patients positive), dimethyloltriazon (10/27 patients positive), melamine-formaldehyde (5/26 patients positive). In these 28 patients also a number of catalysts used in producing these textile finish sporadically were cited positive, *viz.* ammonium chloride, ammonium oxalate and a combination of zinc nitrate with triethylamine hydrochloride. Several of these patients showed a polyvalent sensitivity to finishing compounds of different composition in consequence of which the finding of innocuous clothes became a real problem. As a preliminary conclusion it may be said that in Holland formaldehyde no longer seems to be the main offender, but that a number of reaction products (made from formaldehyde and different other reactants) used for the manufacture of textile finish appear to be the sensitizing substances (*cf.* phenol-formaldehyde shoe adhesive additive, p. 49). Whether these substances must be considered as unreacted intermediate products or as decomposition products (through inappropriate washing procedures) is under investigation.

Whether due to regional differences or due to the fact that the investigations were made during an earlier period, in contradiction to Malten a report of Høvding (1961) mentioned that amongst 2110 routine patch-tested patients during the years 1953 to 1958, 137 cases with formaldehyde-contact hypersensitivity occurred. In 45, this sensitization appeared to be a consequence of textile-finish hypersensitivity. Fisher *et al.* (1962) patch-tested 20 formaldehyde-positive patients with samples of textiles and paper, all containing free formaldehyde, with negative results. Moreover, in a number of cases, the wearing of these textiles gave no untoward effect. Skogh (1959) thought excessive axillary sweating (such as occurs preponderantly in women during puberty, pregnancy and in the menopause) might be a predisposing cause insofar as sweat dissolves the formaldehyde residue from the textile finish, or helps to decompose the finish.

Comparable with regard to the intimacy of the skin contact are the aforementioned cases of hypersensitivity to spectacle resins (Wilde, 1959) and the 4 cases of melamine-resin hypersensitivity observed by Conrad *et al.* (1953) after wearing orthopedic plaster bandages. In soap, urea-formaldehyde resin fillers may be used according to Schneider (1949), who observed a number of contact hypersensitivities due to these resins (but not to formaldehyde). In a brand of nailpolish, a sulfonamide-formaldehyde resin turned out to be the sensitizing component

References p. 54

(Simon 1943). Another brand studied by Keil *et al.* (1944) contained toluenesulfonamide–formaldehyde. In 7 out of 16 patch-tested patients, they found positive reactions to toluenesulfonamide and in 9 out of 21 a hypersensitivity to formaldehyde (all tested patients having shown positive reactions to the resin itself).

Jirásek *et al.* (1961) reported on 41 cases of occupational eczema due to phenoplasts. Patch tests were positive to resol and novolak resins in all patients, whereas tests for phenol and formaldehyde were negative in all instances. Bompart *et al.* (1959) observed allergic skin affections in 16 of 61 workers engaged in the manufacture of scouring paper with a phenol-formaldehyde-resin binder. Hamers (1963) observed *p-tert.*-butylphenol contact hypersensitivity caused by contact with scouring paper or with the binder used to manufacture carborundum grinding stones. Pardon *et al.* (1959) described contact eczema due to phenolformaldehyde-containing glues and varnishes. They observed cases of asthma due to the vapour. Harris (1959) is of opinion that the incidence of contact eczema in plants using formaldehyde-containing resins has gradually been reduced to negligible proportions in recent years, although production has increased by roughly 50%. He thinks there may be a tendency for men who are prone to develop contact eczema (how do they know? K.M.) to seek other employment of their own accord. Phenolformaldehyde resins may be reacted with 1,2-epoxy compounds as described by Havris *et al.* (1954) in the production of plastifiers. Untoward effects are unknown to us.

Celeron, a phenolformaldehyde resin, has been reported to be a potent sensitizer (Queries, 1957). In these cases usually a formaldehyde sensitivity is found. Some phenolformaldehyde resins are so active, that on occasion retention of some of the formaldehyde compounds on a worker's clothes is sufficient to sensitize members of his family at home. There may be further reasons for incomprehensible spread or recurrence of skin manifestations due to formaldehyde or related compounds: Peck *et al.* (1956) considered the use of facial tissue, of which the wet strength had been improved by adding ± 2% urea-formaldehyde or melamine-formaldehyde to the weight of the paper, as a possible cause of contact eczema of the face. With the Draize–Shelanski technique combined with usage test, they found 3 out of 50 volunteers sensitized (usually due to formaldehyde), with positive usage test on the cheek with the resin-containing paper. Rappaport *et al.* (1941) extensively investigated the case of a histological technician (formaldehyde contact) who developed urticaria which started on the second and third fingers of the right hand and on the lips, but later became generalized. Smoking of glycerin-containing cigarettes was the cause of recurrences which were at first not understood. Combustion of glycerine gives rise to acrolein formation. This aldehyde, aliphatic aldehydes up to stearyl aldehyde, citronellal and allylacetaldehyde also gave positive reactions. Contact urticaria case reports are rare, presumably because research in this direction has often been omitted.

SPECIFIC PREVENTION

It may be concluded from the work of Bourret *et al.* (1958) that it might be wise not to employ females between 40 and 60 years of age for work with a formaldehyde risk.

Some of the resin glues are primary skin irritants (Schwartz *et al.* 1943) and these should be handled with gloves. The sleeves should fasten over the gloves at the wrist to prevent irritants from falling into the gloves. If dusts or fumes (phenol, formaldehyde) escape during processing, these should be exhausted from the actual sites of emanation. Warm presses should be exhausted a few minutes before opening and taking the cured articles out. Schwartz *et al.* (1943) advised the use of a mixture of lanoline and castor oil against formaldehyde fumes. Lockey (1944) advised formulae containing 70% alcohol which neutra-

References p. 54

lize phenol and formaldehyde when present on the skin (fire hazard).

If the work is of a varied type, such as the work of a cobbler, Malten (1958) advised that all articles should first be prepared up to the stage where they must be glued. Then, at a fixed time during the working hours, in a more or less separated part of the workshop assigned for this job the glueing of all articles should be done at once. The workman should then wear a special apron and use special tools, both used exclusively for glueing. If uniform articles are to be glued, holders should be constructed to hold the articles in place during application of the adhesive in order to obviate splashing on the skin of the left hand. There should be a hollow space in the surface of cobblers' workbenches into which the soles can be fitted by using a fork. After spreading the glue on with a brush, the soles are lifted out with the same fork.

The Chemical Safety Data Sheets SD-4 (1946) and SD-1 (1952) give extensive information about handling precautions for phenol and formaldehyde. The threshold limit value (MAC) for phenol is given as 5 p.p.m. (= 19 mg/m^3), for formaldehyde as 5 p.p.m. (= 6 mg/m^3) (American Conference Governmental Industrial Hygienists 1962).

REFERENCES

American Conference Governmental Industrial Hygienists, *Threshold Limit Values*, Detroit, Michigan, 1962.

ARCHANGELSKAJA, G. V., *Gigiena Truda i Prof. Zabolevaniya*, 1/4 (1957) 29. Ref.: QUOOSS, 1959.

BAADER, E. W., Investigation of health damages from artificial resins. *Reichsarbeitsbl.*, 3 (1932) 173. Ref.: *U.S. Publ. Health Service*, 1945.

BAADER, E. W. and H. WITTGENS, Gesundheitsgefahren durch Staub im Eisenbahnbetrieb. *Ärztl. Dienst*, 60 (1957) 30.

BANIK, E., Das Formmaskenverfahren nach Croning in der Giessereitechnik unter Berücksichtigung des Arbeits- und Nachbarschutzes. *Zbl. Arbeitsmed.*, 9 (1959) 1.

BERGER, L. B., H. H. SCHRENK, R. W. STEWART, J. A. GALE and L. E. SEIFFERT, Toxicity and flame resistance of thermosetting plastics. *U.S. Dept. of Interior, Bureau of Mines*, 1947, R. I. 4134. Ref.: J. SENDROY *et al.* 1952.

BLOHM, S. G., Formaldehyde-contact dermatitis. *Acta Dermato-Venereol.*, 39 (1959) 450.

BOLTON, K., J. E. CULLINGSWORTH, B. P. GHOSH and J. W. COBB, Primary gaseous products of carbonization. *J. Chem. Soc.*, 1 (1942) 252.

BOMPART, P. V. and G. SMAGGHE, Quelques remarques d'ordre pratique à propos d'une application industrielle des résines formophénolique. *Arch. Maladies Prof.*, 20 (1959) 64.

BOURNE, H. G. and S. SEFERIAN, Insufficiently polymerized resins, used for wrinkle-proofing clothing, may liberate toxic quantities of formaldehyde. *Ind. Med. Surg.*, 28 (1959) 232.

BOURRET, J., F. TOLOT, M. L. POLLET and M. GENEVOIS, Les dermatoses professionnelles provoquées par le formol et ses dérivés industriels. *Arch. Maladies Prof.*, 19 (1958) 611.

BRUNNER, L., Neuere beruflich bedingte Hauterkrankungen. *Berufsdermatosen*, 10 (1962) 61.

Chemical Safety Data Sheet SD-1. *Properties and Essential Information for Safe Handling and Use of Formaldehyde*, Manufact. Chemists' Assoc., Washington, 1952.

Chemical Safety Data Sheet SD-4. *Properties and Essential Information for Safe Handling and Use of Phenol*, Manufact. Chemists' Assoc., Washington, 1946.

COLEMAN, E. H., Gaseous combustion products from plastics. *Plastics*, 24 (1959) 416.

CONRAD, A. H. and L. T. FORD, Allergic contact dermatitis caused by Melmac orthopedic composition. *J. Am. Med. Assoc.*, 153 (1953) 557.

COULANT, P. LE and G. LOPES, L'allergie au formol et à ses dérivés; diagnostic et désensibilisation. *Arch. Maladies Prof.*, 22 (1961) 769.

ELKINS, H. B., *The Chemistry of Industrial Toxicology*, Wiley, New York, 1959.

ETTINGER, J. and M. JEREMIAS, A study of the health hazards involved in working with flameproofed fabrics. *Monthly Rev. Div. Ind. Hyg. N.Y.*, 34 (1955) 25.

FISHER, A. A., N. B. KANOF and E. M. BIONDI, Free formaldehyde in textiles and paper. *Arch. Dermatol.*, 86 (1962) 753.

FOST, J. and N. HJÖRTH, Contact dermatitis from hydrazine hydrochloride in soldering flux; cross-sensitization to apresoline and isoniazid. *Acta Dermato-Venereol.*, 39 (1959) 82.

GAUL, L. E. and G. B. UNDERWOOD, The condensation of phenol and formaldehyde to produce a sensitizer unrelated to the formaldehyde component. *J. Invest. Dermatol.*, 12 (1949) 1.

GLASS, W. I., Outbreak of formaldehyde dermatitis. *New Zealand Med. J.*, 60 (1961) 423. Ref.: *Bull. Hyg.*, 37 (1962) 569.

GIEL, C. P., J. JAMPOL and E. KOEHLER, Health hazards from flameproofed fabrics. *Monthly Rev. Div. Ind. Hyg. N.Y.*, 35 (1956) 20.

HAMERS, A., personal communication (1963).

HANSLIAN, L. and V. ROUS, Causes of health injuries by urea-formaldehyde moulding substance. *Czech. Hyg.*, 3 (1958) 22. Ref.: QUOOSS, 1959.

HARRIS, D. K., Health problems in the manufacture and use of plastics. *Brit. J. Ind. Med.*, 10 (1953) 255.

HARRIS, D. K., Some hazards in the manufacture and use of plastics. *Brit. J. Ind. Med.*, 16 (1959) 221.

HAVRIS, T. G., H. HORNING and H. A. NEVILLE, Résines phenolformaldehyde modifiées aux 1,2-epoxy. *Ind. Plastiques Mod. (Paris)*, 6/12 (1954) 52.

HENSON, V., The toxicity of some aliphatic aldehydes. *J. Occupational Med.*, 1 (1959) 457.

HØVDING, G., Contact eczema due to formaldehyde in resin-finished textiles. *Acta Dermatol.-Venereol.*, 41 (1961) 194.

JIRASEK, L. and R. SCHWANK, Phenolics. *Pracovni Lékar.*, 13/5 (1961) 217. Ref.: *C.I.S.Doc. Dubb Mka* – 2057, 1961.

KEIL, H. and L. VAN DIJCK, Dermatitis due to nail polish with the chief allergic component toluene sulfonamide formaldehyde resin and related substances *A.M.A. Arch. Dermatol. Syphilol.*, 50 (1944) 39.

KEY, M. M., Some unusual allergic reactions in industry. *Arch. Dermatol.*, 83 (1961) 3.

LEFAUX, R., La toxicité des matières plastiques en rapport avec l'hygiène industrielle. *Atti XI. Congresso Intern. Med. del Lavoro, Napoli*, 1 (1954) 83.

LOCKEY, S. D., Contact dermatitis resulting from the manufacture of synthetic resins and methods of control. *J. Allergy*, 15 (1944) 188.

LUDWIG, H., Acute formaldehyde bronchiolitis in workmen handling artificial resin. *Samml. Vergiftungsf.*, 6 (1935) 227. Ref.: *U.S.Publ. Health Service*, 1945.

MALTEN, K. E., *Beroepsekzeem bij het verwerken van kunststoffen*, Thesis, Amsterdam, 1956.

MALTEN, K. E., Occupational eczema due to *p-tert.*-butylphenol in a shoe adhesive. *Dermatologica*, 117 (1958) 103.

MALTEN, K. E., Contacteczeem door industrieel gebruikte hydrazine derivaten met groepsovergevoeligheid voor hydralazine (apresoline) en isoniazide (INH). *Ned. Tijdschr. Geneesk.*, 106 II (1962a) 2219.

MALTEN, K. E., Dermatological aspects of plastics. *Proc. XIIth Intern. Congr. Dermatology, Washington*, 1962b (in press).

MALTEN, K. E., Textile finish contact hypersensitivity. *Arch. Dermatol.*, 88 (1963) to be published.

MARKUSON, K. E., T. F. MANCUSO and J. S. SOET, Dermatitis due to formaldehyde resins. *Ind. Med. Surg.*, 12 (1943) 383.

MORRILL, E. E., Formaldehyde exposure from paper process solved by air sampling and current studies. *Air conditioning, heating, ventilation*, 58 (1961) 94. Ref.: *Publ. Health Eng. Abstr.*, 19/10 (1961) 19.

MOSS, R. H., C. F. JACKSON and J. SEIBERLICH, Toxicity of carbon monoxide and hydrogen cyanide gas mixtures. *Arch. Ind. Hyg.*, 4 (1951) 53.

OETTINGEN, W. F. VON, Phenol and its derivatives. *Natl. Inst. Health, Bull.*, No. 190. G.P.O., Washington, 1949.

PARDON, N. and P. V. BOMPART, Quelques formes cliniques d'intolérance aux résines phénol-formol. *Arch. Maladies Prof.*, 20 (1959) 63.

PECK, S. M. and L. L. PALITZ, Sensitization to facial tissue with urea-formaldehyde resin. *J. Am. Med. Assoc.*, 160 (1956) 1226.

Public Health Service, U.S., Formaldehyde – its toxicity and potential dangers. *Natl. Inst. Health, Publ. Health Rept.*, 1945, Suppl. 181.

Queries and Minor Notes, Celeron. *J. Am. Med. Assoc.* 165 (1957) 642.

QUOOSS, H., *Gesundheitsgefahren in der Kunststoffindustrie*, Barth, Leipzig, 1959.

RAPPAPORT, B. Z. and M. M. HOFFMAN, Urticaria due to aliphatic aldehydes. *J. Am. Med. Assoc.*, 116 (1941) 2656.

Roff, W. J., The determination of the formaldehyde yield of cellulose textiles treated with formaldehyde, urea-formaldehyde or melamine-formaldehyde. *J. Textile Inst.*, 47 (1956) T 309.

Schaefer, W., *Einführung in das Kunststoffgebiet*, Geest & Portig, Leipzig, 1953.

Schneider, W., Zur Frage der Hautverträglichkeit neuartiger Kunstharz-Füllstoffe (Ureum-formaldehyde) für Seifen. *Deut. Med. Wochschr.*, 74 (1949) 741.

Schultheiss, E., Überempfindlichkeit gegenüber Hydrazin. *Berufsdermatosen*, 7 (1959) 131.

Schwartz, L., Dermatitis from new synthetic resin fabric finishes. *J. Invest. Dermatol.*, 4 (1941) 459.

Schwartz, L. and F. Botvinick, Skin hazards in manufacture of glass wool and thread. *Ind. Med.*, 12 (1943) 143.

Schwartz, L., S. Peck and J. Dunn, Dermatitis from resin glue in war industries. *Publ. Health Rept. U.S.*, 58 (1943) 899.

Schwartz, L., L. Tulipan and D. J. Birmingham, *Occupational Diseases of the Skin*, Lea & Febiger, Philadelphia, 1957.

Sendroy, J., J. D. O'Neal and G. C. Pitts, Hazards from thermal decomposition of motor-insulating materials. *Arch. Ind. Hyg.*, 5 (1952) 330.

Simon, F. A., Nail polish eczema. *Southern Med. J.*, 36 (1943) 157.

Skogh, M., Axillary eczema in women, a syndrome. *Acta Dermatol-Venereol.*, 39 (1959) 369.

Tara, S., Intolérance? Sensibilisation? Allergie pulmonaire au formol? *Arch. Maladies Prof.*, 17 (1956) 66.

Tübich, G. E., I. H. Davis and B. D. Bloomfield, Occupational health studies of the shell-molding process. *Arch. Ind. Health*, 21 (1960) 424.

Weger, H., Thalamic symptom complex in formaldehyde poisoning. *Z. Ges. Neurol. Psychiat.*, 111 (1927) 370. Ref.: *U.S. Publ. Health Service*, 1945.

Wilde, H., Brillengestell Dermatitis. *Dermatol. Wochschr.*, 140 (1959) 1089.

Zielhuis, R. L., *Workers in a resin factory*, unpublished investigation, Leiden, 1960.

Zielhuis, R. L., *Asthma by urea-formaldehyde paint*, personal observation, 1961.

6

Alkyd resins

PHYSICO-CHEMICAL PROPERTIES, APPLICATION

Alkyd resins are polycondensates from dicarboxylic acids and polyalcohols; they are a particular type of polyesters, *viz.*: the saturated ones. Because they are chiefly applied as paint vehicles, they are mostly modified with fatty acids (drying or non-drying oils). As dicarboxylic acid, chiefly phthalic acid anhydride (*o*-benzene dicarboxylic acid anhydride) is used; in some cases the unsaturated maleic acid anhydride (ethene dicarboxylic acid anhydride) is added in small quantities. As polyalcohols, mainly glycerol and in some cases pentaerythritol, dipentaerythritol or sorbitol are applied.

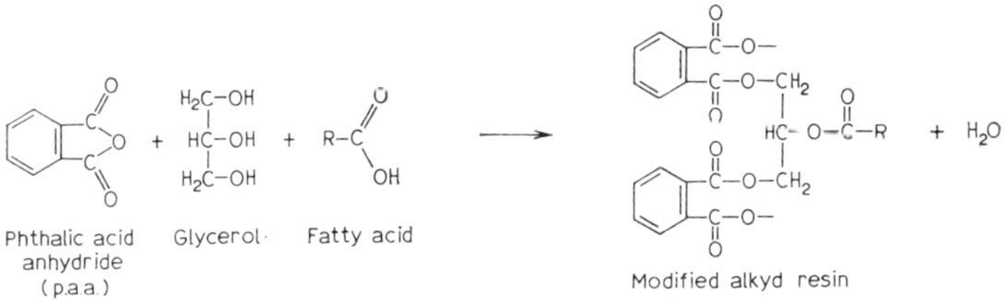

Non-modified alkyd resins may be used as plastifiers; in this case adipic acid, sebacic acid, hexanetriol and butanetriol may also be used as modifying the alcohol component. Of the above-mentioned compounds only the dicarboxylic acids involve in-

References p. 68

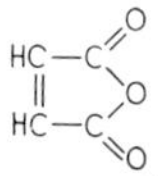

Maleic acid anhydride
(m.a.a.)

dustrial health hazards. Although maleic acid anhydride is mainly used in unsaturated polyesters (see p. 71), in this chapter the properties of both phthalic acid anhydride (p.a.a.) and maleic acid anhydride (m.a.a.) will be discussed because of the similarity of their chemical and biological effects.

Baader (1955), Menschik (1955) and Merlevede *et al.* (1957) described the hygiene of the production of p.a.a. and m.a.a. Because of the increasing application of alkyd resins and unsaturated polyesters since the second world war, huge quantities of both compounds are being produced. P.a.a. is formed by catalytic (V_2O_5) oxidation of naphthalene. The resulting p.a.a. must be gathered from condensation chambers; the exposure to the compounds presents a real hazard. Several impurities may complicate the industrial pathology. Non-purified naphthalene may contain phenols, pyridine, anthracene, carbazol, phenanthrene, pyrocatechin; purification (up to 98%) takes place by melting and distillation. During the oxidation into p.a.a. several by-products may be formed: m.a.a., CO, naphthoquinone. Non-purified p.a.a. still contains 0.5% m.a.a. and 0.1–0.5% naphthoquinone; it is purified by refining and distilling at 200°; purified p.a.a. contains less than 0.1% m.a.a. and 0.001% naphthoquinone. In some factories mercury is used as heat-transferring material. Moreover cracking of naphthalene may yield benzene and –CN compounds (from N-containing impurities).

M.a.a. is produced in a closed system by oxidation of benzene in the presence of V_2O_5; the material is dehydrated by toluene. Exposure to m.a.a., CO, benzene and toluene may therefore exist.

The above-mentioned impurities and by-products (*e.g.* benzene, CO) will not be discussed because these industrial hazards are well known. The glycols are discussed in Chapter 7.

EXPERIMENTAL TOXICOLOGY AND DERMATOLOGY

Exposure of rats and rabbits to 10 g p.a.a./m^3, 4 h per day for several days, interfered with normal breathing; 25% of the animals died. Cats exposed to 3.7 g/m^3, 6 h per day for 7 days, became drowsy; vomiting and anorexia occurred: liver and kidney disease were observed (Gloxhuber; Flury *et al.*, cited by Baader 1955). Policard *et al.* (1949) exposed rats to 'high' concentrations of p.a.a. Reversible congestion and hypersecretion of the mucosae resulted, with obliteration of some bronchioli leading to obstructive emphysema. After one week, however, the lungs were normal again without any residual effects. According to these authors, p.a.a. particularly attacks the upper air passages, as does phthalic acid; only a minor quantity reaches the bronchioli and alveoli. Friebel *et al.* (1956) exposed guinea pigs to dusts and vapours of purified p.a.a., non-purified batches of K7 (98.5% p.a.a., 1% naphthoquinone, 0.5% m.a.a.) or K2 (99.6% p.a.a., 0.3% naphthoquinone, 0.1% m.a.a.). Exposure of guinea pigs to dust (p.a.a.: 8.5 mg/m^3; K2:66 mg/m^3; K7:55 mg/m^3; 3 h per day; periods of 4-days inhalation – 10 days rest; total 8 months) caused hyperemia of mucosae and secondary pneumonitis. Exposure to vapour (p.a.a.: 614.5 mg/m^3; K2:1297 mg/m^3; K7:947 mg/m^3; 30 min per day; 4–8 days) resulted in decreased respiration rate, increased nasal secretion with loosening of mucosae and (peri)bronchitis. The authors' suggestion that K2 and K7 vapour possessed greater toxicity than purified p.a.a. does not seem to be valid because the concentrations were not equivalent. The oral lethal dose for rats was 2.5–5 g/kg, the same for the three mentioned batches; these animals died from tubular necrosis of the kidney. In the above-mentioned experiments with inhalation of sometimes very high concentrations of p.a.a., the main signs of toxicity were due to revers-

References p. 68

ible irritation of the epithelium of the respiratory tract; systemic toxicity by resorption seemed to be of much less importance. In some experimental exposures to p.a.a. (Kühnl 1951) or m.a.a. (guinea pigs, above 1.9 mg/m^3 for 1 h; Tanaka 1956) keratitis corneae was noted.

INDUSTRIAL TOXICOLOGY

Baader (1955) examined 14 workers, exposed to p.a.a. and accumulated information from factories producing p.a.a. and m.a.a. in several European countries. He listed the following symptoms:

- Irritation of the eyes, without corneal defects.
- Irritation of the mucosae of nose (and sinus), larynx, trachea and bronchi, sometimes with epistaxis, hemoptysis, asthma.
- Anorexia, gastric complaints, asthenia, cachexia.
- Erythema, eczema, burns, urticaria.

Baader himself indicated the possibility of toxic effects caused by the impurities. Exposure to impure p.a.a. for instance was more likely to give rise to asthma, rhinitis and gastralgia than exposure to the purified materials. Many workers got 'brown hands', due to naphthoquinone. According to Baader the MAC should be below 25 mg p.a.a./m^3, because at 25 mg/m^3 he still observed irritation of mucosae and one case of asthma. This experience is probably based upon non-purified p.a.a. Menschik (1955), who himself reacted to inhalation of p.a.a. with asthma and/or urticaria, examined 71 workers, who were exposed for less than 20 months. In addition to the above-mentioned symptoms, he also observed slight anemia, leucocytosis and reticulocytosis, decreased Ca-level in blood, disturbed serum-protein pattern, positive Rumpel–Leeds, high reflexes, hypotension and many non-specific feelings of ill-health. According to Menschik, all the effects described were due to p.a.a.; in addition he mentioned the possibility of other effects caused by naphthalene, Hg, V_2O_5, CO, benzene, –CN. Although Menschik's investigations were very extensive, he did not examine control groups; the significance of some biochemical data and of some non-specific symptoms has not been proved adequately. According to Frede (1962) the hygienic problems in Menschik's factory disappeared after taking technical preventive measures. Merlevede *et al.* (1957) took up a strong position against Baader and Menschik. Many of the above-mentioned effects were supposed to be due to impurities and by-products. In their opinion, p.a.a. intoxication has a more uniform pattern with less systemic effects. Merlevede *et al.* came to these conclusions after investigations in some Belgian factories. They examined 23 workers exposed, among others, to non-purified naphthalene, some of them for 25 years; they only noted one case of eczema, and no other effects. Pressing of this material caused slight irritation of the conjunctivae. Gathering p.a.a. from the condensation chambers resulted in the above-mentioned irritative effects, but many so-called p.a.a. effects were supposed to be due to V_2O_5: pallor of the skin, discoloration of the tongue, attacks of coughing with hemoptysis, dyspnoea, thoracic pains, tremor, bronchospasm, bronchitis, hypertension. M.a.a. is reported to be more aggressive than p.a.a., although for 15 years no serious intoxication was observed by Merlevede *et al.* in 12 exposed workers. M.a.a. is more readily converted into the aggressive maleic acid by atmospheric H_2O, and the melting point of m.a.a. is considerably lower than that of p.a.a.: 53° *versus* 132°. Kapustkina *et al.* (1959) reported data from a Russian factory. They examined 118 workers exposed to the following atmospheric concentrations: 10–18 mg p.a.a./m^3, 0.27–0.57 mg naphthoquinone/m^3, 30–180 mg CO/m^3. More than half of these workers registered recurring bronchitis, 21% of them recurring gastritis and 16% chronic rhinopharyngitis; the blood pressure was generally decreased; numerous neurovegetative symptoms were noted (exposure to CO?). They suggested a MAC of 10 mg p.a.a./m^3. Donnat (1944), Bénard *et al.* (1945), Roche (1947), Policard (1949), Bourret *et al.*

References p. 68

(1950) and Munari *et al.* (1960), recording their experiences in French and Italian industries, stressed the preponderance of irritative effects on the respiratory tract (among others asthma), but they reported in addition more general symptoms of ill-health. Frede (1962) examined 118 workers, many of them exposed for more than 10 years. He found a definitely increased incidence of bronchitis with or without emphysema (cumulative effect), reversible conjunctivitis, and some cases of contact dermatitis. According to Frede, the respiratory symptoms were the result of primary irritation, and not of allergy.

Kern (1939) reported a case of allergic asthma in a chemist in the painting industry; a rhinitis preceded the asthma. A scratch test with p.a.a. crystals and with p.a.a. 1 : 1000 in alcohol was strongly positive: a positive Prausnitz–Küstner test proved the allergic basis.

Merlevede *et al.* (1957) considered the hazard in departments producing phthalate esters as practically non-existent. Irritation of eyes and air passages, even slight bronchitis, in workers employed for 2 years in the production of octyl- and butyl-phthalates, was reported, however, by Pisani (1960).

The Dutch Labour Inspectorate (1960) reported a chemical bronchitis in a worker exposed to m.a.a. vapour from a reaction kettle. Zielhuis (1960) examined 37 workers in a synthetic resin factory, employed for at least 2 years (see p. 44). Several workers reported attacks of laryngitis, pharyngitis and conjunctivitis after accidental exposures to flakes or vapours of p.a.a. and m.a.a.; no residual effects on the air passages and lungs were observed, nor disturbances of liver, blood or kidney.

In 265 workers from printing shops, exposed to m.a.a., Tanaka (1956) observed 17 cases of superficial keratitis; most of the workers complained of eye irritation. The consequences of an accident while unloading m.a.a.-containing casks were reported by Russo *et al.* (1959); from the workers exposed to m.a.a. dust, 7 subjects developed severe conjunctivitis and bronchitis, which healed without residual effects.

Even purified p.a.a. may contain small quantities of m.a.a. and very small quantities of naphthoquinones, according to Merlevede *et al.* (1957). Naphthoquinones give rise to a red to brown discoloration of the wet skin due to a chemical binding with components of the deeper layers of the skin. For that reason this discoloration cannot be washed away and only clears after a delay of three weeks or more by shedding the coloured layer. Presumably due to this binding capacity, naphthoquinones may also act as contact sensitizers giving rise to contact eczema. Moreover these substances are keratoplastic and this may be the reason of the oil acne-like manifestations sometimes observed (Menschik 1955).

P.a.a. and m.a.a., if cold, are not very harmful to a dry skin (hot compounds may cause burns). On a sweating skin, however, both substances are hydrated to the corresponding acids and these act as caustics causing dermatitis and first- or second-degree burns. M.a.a. is more dangerous in this respect than p.a.a. because it readily takes up water from the atmosphere, thus converting more quickly into the acid than p.a.a. Whether skin resorption of p.a.a. or p.a. is possible or not is not cited in the literature, but may be concluded from an observation made by Menschick (1955), who observed an itching urticarial exanthema on the skin outside the gasmask. Baader (1955) and Menschick (1955) both mentioned true allergic urticaria and contact eczema due to p.a.a. or p.a. without citing testing concentrations. However Kern (1939) investigating a case of p.a. asthma, observed in his patient a positive cutis reaction on 1/1000 p.a. dissolved in alcohol, whereas controls remained negative. The reaction of Prausnitz–Küstner was also positive. Kühnl (1951), being an engineer, reported on phthalic acid diethyl ester causing dermatitis and contact eczema, on phthalic acid dibutyl ester causing dermatitis and on phthalic acid diamyl ester causing both dermatitis and contact eczema. Skin

References p. 68

resorption of the first named substance is possible, and may cause the appearance of p.a. in the urine.

Impurities of maleic acid anhydride may be, among others, maleic acid and fumaric acid (Merlevede *et al.* 1957).

Investigating men who worked with unsaturated polyester resins, Malten (1956) patch-tested with phthalic acid (5% in water) and maleic acid (0.5% in water). Neither of these substances gave a positive patch test in persons sensitized to the resin, but fumaric acid patch tests (testing conc. pure) showed positive results in two of these men, and phthalic acid anhydride in one (see Table 1, p. 79). Wondering whether esters of maleic acid would have acted as sensitizer in these men, he wanted to establish and to control the patch-testing concentration of diethyl ester of maleic acid (0.5% in alcohol). After he himself had reacted negatively, he applied patch tests on volunteers: 6 engineers in the firm where he carried out the investigation. Although only one of these engineers had a contact eczema (not due to polyester resins), he observed 4 positive allergic reactions after 24 hours contact with diethyl ester of maleic acid. These engineers may thus have been primarily sensitized through the patch-testing procedure, which is an extremely rare occurrence. Nevertheless, caution should be taken in patch-testing with this substance, as it may be one of the small number of known primary sensitizers marked in the list of Schwartz *et al.* (1957). Finally, Malten desires to report the case of a female laboratory worker engaged in synthesizing semi-stearate of maleic acid anhydride who became contact-sensitized to this substance on the ninth day of her experiments.

Owada (1954) used as patch-testing concentration 0.07% maleic acid anhydride in (water-free) adeps lanae recently prepared.

Schwartz (1943) reported on an outbreak of contact eczema from hair lacquers, composed of combinations of rosin and maleic acid anhydride, and one of the two also containing ethylene glycol (and thus possibly giving rise to the formation of polyester macromolecules). Rosin chiefly consists of abietic acid and it is a known sensitizer. As no patch tests were made with the separate ingredients, the sensitizing substance in these lacquers remains unknown.

Klauder (1948) reported contact eczema from 'Scottissue' towels localized on hands, arms and face due to a special finish on paper towels. This contained the diethylene glycol ester maleic anhydride adduct. Wet patch tests with the towel paper and with ordinary manilla packing paper were positive.

Schwartz *et al.* (1957) mentioned the occurrence of (contact?) dermatitis in the use of alkyd resins for laminating wood and fabrics. Dioctylphthalate and butylbenzylphthalate are irritants, moreover dioctylphthalate is known as a sensitizer (Lefaux 1955). Malten has recorded one case of contact hypersensitivity to dioctyl phthalate (*cf.* Table 1, p. 79).

NAPHTHALENE

Due to the fact that exposure to naphthalene might easily occur in the production department of p.a.a., the toxicological data will be reviewed here in short (Gerarde 1960):

- Dermatoses, through primary irritation and hypersensitivity.
- Irritation of the eyes.
- General symptoms of headache, sickness, profuse perspiration.
- In high exposure: vomiting, optical neuritis, hematuria, edema, and after 5 years at the least opacities of the eye lens.

In p.a.a. factories only irritation of the eyes has as yet been reported. Gerarde suggested a MAC of 25 p.p.m. (131 mg/m^3).

SPECIFIC PREVENTION

Preventive measures against the hazard from phthalic acid anhydride and maleic acid anhydride should be applied particularly in the production departments of these compounds and in the

References p. 68

early phases of production of alkyd resins. Local and general exhaust ventilation will often be necessary. Contact of the skin especially with hot materials should be avoided. Attention should be paid to the possible occurrence of many toxic by-products. If possible, the monomers should be handled and transported as pastes. Contaminated eyes should be rinsed with weak $CaCO_3$ or NaOH solution. The *Chemical Safety Data Sheet* SD-61 (1956) gives extensive information on first aid and technical preventive measures regarding p.a.a., the *Data Sheet* SD-88 (1962) provides similar information with regard to m.a.a.

Only tentative threshold limits for p.a.a. and m.a.a. have been suggested by some authors; it seems reasonable to keep the p.a.a. level below 10–20 mg/m^3, and the m.a.a. level below 5 mg/m^3.

REFERENCES

BAADER, E. W., Erkrankungen durch Phthalsäure und ihre Verbindungen. *Arch. Gewerbepathol. Gewerbehyg.*, 13 (1955) 419.

BERNARD, E. and M. MARCHAND, Intoxication par l'anhydride phthalique. *Arch. Inst. Méd. Lég. Soc. Lille*, 1945. Ref.: BAADER, 1955.

BOURRET, J., G. GAUTHIER and L. ROCHE, Intoxication par l'anhydride phthalique. *Acta Méd. Lég. Soc. Liège*, 3 (1950) 33.

Chemical Safety Data Sheet SD-61, *Phthalic Anhydride*, Manufact. Chemists' Assoc., Washington, 1956.

Chemical Safety Data Sheet SD-88, *Maleic acid anhydride*, Manufact. Chemists' Assoc., Washington, 1962.

DONNAT, L., Syndrome d'irritation des voies aëriennes supérieures et bronchiques par l'anhydride phthalique. *Méd. Travail*, 2 (1944) 109. Ref.: BAADER, 1955.

Dutch Labour Inspectorate (Arbeidsinspectie), *Ann. Rept.* 1959, The Hague, 1960, p. 125.

FREDE, F., Gesundheitliche Gefahren bei der Herstellung von Phthalsäureanhydrid. *Z. Hyg.*, 3 (1962) 177.

FRIEBEL, H., E. GROSS, L. IMMISCH-SEEHAUSEN, K. H. LINKE and

S. SOMMER, Zur Toxicität von reinem Phthalsäureanhydrid und Rohprodukten, aus der industriellen Phthalsäuresynthese. *Arch. Gewerbepathol. Gewerbehyg.*, 14 (1956) 465.

GERARDE, H. W., *Toxicology and Biochemistry of Aromatic Hydrocarbons*, Elsevier, Amsterdam, 1960.

KAPUSTKINA, T. W., M. S. MENDLIN, A. A. N. NIKITENKO, L. K. SANNIKOVA and B. F. CHIMECZENKO, Die Arbeitsplatzbedingungen und der Gesundheitszustand der Arbeiter bei der Herstellung von Phthalsäureanhydrid. *Gigiena Truda i Prof. Zabolevaniya*, 3 (1959) 28. Ref.: *Zbl. Arbeitsmed.*, 10 (1960) 150.

KERN, R. A., Asthma and allergic rhinitis due to sensitization to phthalic anhydride. *J. Allergy*, 10 (1939) 164.

KLAUDER, J. V., Sensitization dermatitis from 'Scottissue' towels. *A.M.A. Arch. Dermatol. Syphilol.*, 57 (1948) 414.

KÜHNL, O., *Die Schädigungen durch Arbeit*, Bd. 2, Springer, Wien, 1951, p. 160. Ref.: BAADER, 1955.

LEFAUX, R., La toxicologie des matières plastiques en rapport avec l'hygiène industrielle. *Arch. Maladies Prof.*, 16 (1955) 554.

MALTEN, K. E., *Beroepsekseem bij het verwerken van kunststoffen*, Thesis, Amsterdam, 1956.

MENSCHICK, H., Gesundheitliche Gefahren bei der Herstellung von Phthalsäureanhydrid. *Arch. Gewerbepathol. Gewerbehyg.*, 13 (1955) 454.

MERLEVEDE, E., and J. ELSKENS, Les intoxications dues à l'anhydride phthalique, l'anhydride maléique et aux phthalates. *Arch. Belges Méd. Soc.*, 15 (1957) 445.

MUNARI, M. and V. TINAZZI, Aspects of the pathology from exposure to phthalic anhydride. *Rass. Med. Ind.*, 29 (1960) 107. Ref.: *Bull. Hyg.*, 36 (1961) 31.

OWADA, K., N. IDA, C. NAKAGAWA and T. YAMAMOTO, Läppchentest mit Maleinsäure-anhydrid. *J. Osaka City Med. Centre*, 3 (1954) 269. Ref.: *Berufsdermatosen*, 4 (1956) 154.

PISANI, F., Pathology of the workers employed in the preparation of octyl- and butyl-phthalates. *Med. Lavoro*, 51 (1960) 107. Ref.: *Bull. Hyg.*, 35 (1960) 972.

POLICARD, A., G. GAUTHIER, R. HUGONNIER and L. ROCHE, L'intoxication par l'anhydride phthalique. *Arch. Maladies Prof.*, 10 (1949) 70.

ROCHE, J., *Les accidents causés par l'anhydride phthalique dans l'industrie*, Thesis, Paris, 1947. Ref.: BAADER, 1955.

RUSSO, L. and D. ZANNINI, Akute Gruppenvergiftung mit Maleinsäure-anhydrid. *Folia Med.*, 62 (1959) 35. Ref.: *Zbl. Arbeitsmed.*, 11 (1961) 91.

SCHWARTZ, L., An outbreak of dermatitis from hair lacquer. *Publ. Health Rept. U.S.*, 58 (1943) 44.

SCHWARTZ, L., L. TULIPAN and D. J. BIRMINGHAM, *Occupational Diseases of the Skin*, Lea & Febiger, Philadelphia, 1957.

TANAKA, S., Lesion of the eye caused by maleic anhydride vapour. *J. Sci. Labour*, 32 (1956) 117. Ref.: *Bull. Hyg.*, 31 (1956) 839.

ZIELHUIS, R. L., Unpublished investigation, Leiden, 1960.

7

Unsaturated polyesters

PHYSICO-CHEMICAL PROPERTIES, APPLICATION

Generally, plastics are not suitable as such for the construction of large rigid bodies. The mechanical strength may, however, be considerably increased by reinforcing the plastics in a way more or less similar to the reinforcing of concrete with iron rods or wire-netting. Glass-fibre material (see p. 194) is generally used for this purpose, while the plastics serve as binding compounds. The following plastics are applied as such: unsaturated polyesters, epoxy resins (see p. 102) and pheno- or aminoplasts (see p. 40). In addition, the following auxiliary compounds may be used in one of the stages of processing: pigments (generally non-toxic), fillers (such as crystalline or amorphous silica, p. 204), solvents (among others trichloroethylene, turpentine, methylene chloride, methyl ethyl ketone, acetone, toluene), parting compounds (either wax or polyvinylalcohol solutions).

In this chapter special attention will be paid to the unsaturated polyesters. These resins are built from bifunctional organic acids and diols; one of the components carries an unsaturated bond. The unsaturated polyesters are high-molecular linear syrupy products. As bifunctional acids, especially the unsaturated maleic acid anhydride (see p. 60) is used, whereas phthalic acid anhydride (see p. 60) may be added in varying amounts. By using anhydrides the production of a by-product (H_2O) in these polycondensation reactions is avoided. As diols, generally,

References p. 82

diethylene glycol (2,2-oxydiethanol) or 1,2-propylene glycol (1,2-propanediol) are applied.

The polyester resins are processed as solution in styrene (vinylbenzene), about 65% resin to 35% solvent.

The viscous unsaturated linear polyesters are cured by means of *cross-linking agents*, which link the unsaturated bonds (polymerization reaction, see p. 2). In most cases styrene may be used for this purpose, serving at the same time as solvent and as curing agent. In a minority of cases diallyl phthalate or triallyl cyanurate, both of them carrying unsaturated allyl bonds, are applied as cross-linking agent. In order to start the cross-linking polymerization reaction, small amounts of catalysts have to be added: organic peroxides (see p. 211). Accelerators, usually Co-octoate, Co-stearate, Co-naphthenate or dimethylaniline are needed to promote the catalytic reactions.

Of the compounds mentioned above, styrene is being applied in large amounts. It is a volatile (b.p. 145.2°; v.p. 4.3 mm Hg at 15°) liquid. Exposure, either by inhalation or by skin contact, readily occurs.

From the viewpoint of hygiene, the techniques of processing reinforced plastics are of considerable importance. The *hand-lay-up* procedure is most frequently used: glass-fibre material is spread into a mould and impregnated with polyester and styrene (after adding the various auxiliary compounds). Impregnation takes place by means of tamponing with a brush and rolling with metal rollers. This work is called 'laminating'. If the moulds are large (boats, yachts, car bodies), the evaporation area of the volatile styrene is extensive. The working postures are sometimes bad (bending, kneeling, squatting). The hand-lay-up method involves intensive manual contact. The end-product often has to be finished by sawing, fraising, cutting, planing, creating a polyester–glass fibre dust (see p. 195). In the series production of smaller objects mechanized techniques may be applied: suction of the glass fibres unto a perforated mould followed by curing of the polyester under pressure at increased temperatures. In recent years, winding and spraying techniques have come into use.

The hazard of inhaling styrene is particularly great when applying the hand-lay-up technique in the construction of large bodies. According to Hartogensis (1962) the styrene content in atmospheric air in production departments of small objects was well below 100 p.p.m., generally in the order of 30–70 p.p.m., but in the construction of yachts (length up to 12 m) this concentration could easily go up to 300 or 400 p.p.m., particularly during the assembling of prefabricated body elements. Rogers (1955) mentioned concentrations of 200–700 p.p.m. during the mixing of the components (exothermic reaction) and during lamination work in constructing plastic swimming pools. Stephenson *et al.* (1960) measured concentrations of 200–700 p.p.m. during spraying or brushing of anticorrosion isopolyesters (on *m*-phthalic acid basis). Evaporation of styrene occurs not only during the laminating procedure, but also during the curing of the impregnated mass. Tuchenko *et al.* (1961) determined an evaporation of 4.5 g styrene/m^2/min during laminating, and 1.7 g/m^2/min directly thereafter; even after 24 h styrene was still measurable in the air. Hess (1959) reported much lower values: 11 g/m^2/h during curing; Rogers (1955) mentioned the same order of magnitude: 5 g/sq.ft./h. These values will vary according to the type of the polyester–styrene mixture.

Methods for the determination of styrene in air have been described by Rowe *et al.* (1943), Zawadzki (1961) and Hartogensis (1962).

EXPERIMENTAL TOXICOLOGY AND DERMATOLOGY

Styrene

In laboratory experiments (Spencer *et al.* 1942), rats survived exposure to 1300 p.p.m. for 30 h, to 2500 p.p.m. for 8 h, and to 10,000 p.p.m. for 1 h. All rats died when they were exposed to these concentrations for 40, 21 or 3 h respectively. Guinea

References p. 82

pigs were more sensitive. The animals either died from narcosis (primary lethality) or from severe irritation of the respiratory tract (secondary lethality). Repeated exposure to 1300 p.p.m. for 7–8 h per day, 5 days per week was tolerated by rats without definite toxic effects for 6 months, by rabbits and monkeys for 12 months. Disturbances of the hemopoietic system were not observed; sometimes dubious and slight liver degeneration occurred. Guinea pigs were more sensitive; they tolerated an exposure to 650 p.p.m. for 6 months. Rylova (1955), who also examined the higher nervous activity, noted some effects in rabbits exposed to 55–435 p.p.m. Young rats, exposed to 750 p.p.m. 3 h per day, for 27 days, proved to be incapacitated in swimming tests. The LD_{50}-oral for rats was 5.0 g/kg (Wolf *et al.* 1956). The effective acute toxicity in white mice (inhalation 45 mg/l for 2 lots) was for benzene 11.5 times the e.a.t. for styrene (Pokrowsky 1961).

Spencer *et al.* (1942) concluded from their experiments that an exposure to 400 p.p.m. would not result in serious health hazards or discomfort. Concentrations beyond 600 p.p.m. had an immediate irritating effect with increased nasal secretions, whereas also exposure to 200–400 p.p.m. was very disagreeable because of the odour. According to Wolf *et al.* (1956), exposure to 100 p.p.m. was tolerable; concentrations of 60 p.p.m. did not irritate; the odour threshold, however, was below 10 p.p.m. Exposure to increasing concentrations up to 1100 p.p.m. for 1 h resulted in severe lachrymation, increased nasal secretion, feeling of a felt-like tongue, and uncertain gait (Kalsbeek *et al.* 1960). One gets quickly accustomed to the odour and the irritating properties of styrene (Eich 1960), except in high concentrations.

Several investigators established the absence of effects on hematopoiesis in chronic experiments (Spencer *et al.* 1942; Loeser *et al.* 1956; Wolf *et al.* 1956; Hofmann 1961). Only Pokrowsky (1961) mentioned an instability in the number of leucocytes in rabbits, but no leucopenia after chronic inhalation of 0.8 mg/h. Styrene proved to be irritating to rabbits' skin, particularly after repeated application; the effect was comparable to the effect of toluene or benzene (Spencer *et al.* 1942).

From the experiments mentioned above it may be concluded that styrene has moderate narcotic properties, whereas the odour and the strong irritative properties provide a good warning signal against excessive dangerous concentrations; chronic effects on liver, kidney or bone marrow have not been observed. A MAC of 100 p.p.m. (420 mg/m^3) has been suggested by the American Conference of Governmental Industrial Hygienists (1962), predominantly based upon the irritative properties.

Allyl compounds

Very few experimental data have been reported on diallyl phthalate and triallyl cyanurate. The volatility is low. The possibility of percutaneous resorption has not been investigated. The allyl group has well-known toxic properties; exposure to allyl alcohol and allyl chloride resulted in degeneration of liver and kidney (Dunlap *et al.* 1958; Torkelson *et al.* 1959a, 1959b). The LD_{50}-oral for diallylphthalate for rabbits is 1679 mg/kg (Spector 1956). Detoxication of the cross-linking agents in the body may possibly give rise to the formation of other allyl compounds. According to Hagen (1956) triallyl cyanurate possesses irritative properties for skin and eyes; oral intake of 250 mg/kg was said to cause slight disturbances of the nervous system in experimental animals.

Glycols

Diethylene glycol and propylene glycol, both used as alcohol components for the polyester resins, possess a very low volatility. Diethylene glycol is very toxic, particularly in regard to the kidneys (formation of oxalic acids). A potential industrial hazard exists. Propylene glycol does not possess this effect; it is a rather harmless compound (Browning 1953, 1959). Triethylene glycol also possesses a low toxicity.

References p. 82

Catalysts and accelerators

The hygienic properties of organic peroxides have been discussed elsewhere (see p. 211). Dimethylaniline may be resorbed through the skin; it has toxic properties similar to those of aniline.

INDUSTRIAL TOXICOLOGY

Rogers (1955) described 'styrene sickness': nausea, vomiting, anorexia, asthenia. This occurred in workers exposed to 200–700 p.p.m. styrene during laminating and mixing operations in the construction of polyester swimming pools. The symptoms always disappeared within a few hours after interruption of work. In workers exposed to an average concentration of about 50 p.p.m. Bardodej *et al.* (1960) only noted increased lassitude and drowsiness in comparison to non-exposed workers; at the end of the working day the excretion of benzoic acid amounted to 100–2200 mg/l. These authors suggest 50 p.p.m. (210 mg/m^3) as maximum acceptable concentration.

The results of investigations, performed in Holland in the years 1960–1962 in some reinforced-polyester industries, particularly making polyester yachts (length 8–12 m), were reported by Kalsbeek *et al.* (1960), Jongh (1962), Hartogensis (1962), Zielhuis (1962a, 1962b) and Winsemius (1962). Physical examination of 70 exposed workers did not reveal any occupational pathology. In 18 workers exposed to concentrations beyond 100 p.p.m. styrene, more a-specific symptoms were noted than in 34 workers exposed to 30–70 p.p.m.; the latter group did not differ from a non-exposed control group of 18 workers. The first group mentioned an increased incidence of lassitude, gastric disturbances, decreased appetite, headache, dizziness, increased perspiration, drowsiness, irritation of mucosae. The symptoms usually disappeared before starting work again the next day; signs of chronic intoxication were not established. Sickness absenteeism had not increased. Some workers showed an evident correlation between the number of symptoms and the styrene concentration on different days. The overall level of symptoms, however, was probably also dependent on subjective factors such as motivation, eagerness to report symptoms, etc. The authors concluded from these investigations that an exposure to maximal 100 p.p.m. did not guarantee freedom from lighter symptoms related with work (discomfort). A maximum concentration of 50–70 p.p.m. (210–300 mg/m^3) would probably offer greater protection. When constructing large objects, such a concentration, however, can only be reached by intensive local ventilation. Klimkova-Deutschova (1962) suggested a still lower maximum allowable value. She examined 35 workers in two factories, exposed to 183–556 mg/m^3 or 80–417 mg/m^3 for an average of 1.9 years (maximal 3 yrs.) This author not only mentioned a high frequency of a-specific symptoms, but also stressed the occurrence of signs of disturbance of the central and peripheral nervous system. The symptomatology was similar to that of a group of workers exposed to benzene (except the blood dyscrasia) or methylene chloride, but of a less serious character. The total number of exposed workers however, was not given; the high frequency of reported symptoms and signs was not related to the population at risk. Moreover, most of the workers were women beyond the age of 50 years, and a control group not exposed to solvents was not examined. Pokrowsky (1961) reported similar experiences from observation of about 300 workers, mostly female, exposed to concentrations below 600 mg/m^3: disturbances in higher nervous activity, gynecological disorders, instability of the blood count. He even proposed a lowering of the official Russian MAC of 12.5 p.p.m. (50 mg/m^3). (See chapter 10).

The toxicological aspects of other materials used in the processing of reinforced polyesters have been discussed elsewhere (glass-fibre materials, peroxides). Dimethylaniline and Co compounds are used in relatively small amounts; toxicological hazards have not been reported.

References p. 82

Because the uncured unsaturated polyester resin is made by polycondensation of dibasic acid anhydrides with diols, one may expect contact eczemas in workers laminating these resins who have intimate skin contact with these viscous liquids.

Lieber (1955) classified polyester resins as sensitizers. Stephenson *et al.* (1960) did not report sensitizations in the use of isopolyesters. Klauder (1948) observed sensitization dermatitis from 'Scottissue' towels which had been prepared with diethylene glycol ester of 'abalyn' maleic anhydride adduct. Malten (1956) observed 5 patients with contact eczema and positive patch tests to unsaturated polyester resins in a group of 30 workers of an airplane factory. These sensitizations occurred during the first months these resins were in use. The workers were still unskilled, no precautions were taken and the production had scarcely passed the experimental phase. Four of these five patients showed a polysensitization: they showed positive patch tests not only to the resins themselves, but also to various ingredients. Three others engaged in the same glass-fibre laminating work showed a contact hypersensitivity not due to the resins, but only due to various ingredients occurring in this type of work (accelerator, plasticizer, catalyst), see Table 1.

Although contact sensitization to ethylene glycol has been described by Howell (1946), in our investigation none of the tested workers reacted to the ethylene glycol and diethylene glycol. With regard to the acid anhydrides from which the investigated polyester resins were made, we did not find positive patch tests to maleic acid anhydride, and only one + reaction to phthalic acid anhydride (*cf.* Chapter 6, p. 60). According to Feuer *et al.* (1954), maleic acid anhydride is converted to fumaric acid anhydride during polycondensation. This may account for the two positive patch tests with fumaric acid. According to Müller (1954) adipic acid may be built in the polyester resin macromolecule to lessen the brittleness. The cited positive

TABLE 1

RESULTS OF PATCH TESTS WITH UNSATURATED POLYESTER INGREDIENTS

	Patient No. 1	2	3	4	5	6	7	8
Lamellon 6	×	+++	–	×	×	–	–	–
Lamellon 23	++	++	×	+	++	–	–	–
Markon 9	+++	+++	+++	+	–	–	–	–
Bakelite SK 17449	+	+++	×	–	–	–	–	–
Co-naphthenate	–	–	–	–	–	–	++	++
Benzoylperoxide paste	–	++	–	–	++	–	–	++
Cyclohexanone hydroperoxide	–	–	++	++	–	–	–	–
Methyl ethyl ketone hydroperoxide	–	–	–	–	–	–	–	++
Dimethyl phtalate	–	–	–	–	–	++	–	–
Dioctyl phtalate	–	–	–	–	–	–	++	–
Adipic acid	–	++	–	–	–	–	–	–
Fumaric acid	–	+	–	+++	–	–	–	–
Phthalic acid anhydride	–	–	–	–	+	–	–	–

×: no test performed.

reaction to this substance occurred in a research worker, who might have handled this substance separately in experimental work.

A Co-naphthenate contact hypersensitivity was observed twice in this series of patients, whereas dimethylaniline scored no untoward reactions (for peroxides see Chapter 16, p. 211).

After this initial phase, not one polyester resin sensitization has been observed in a survey in the following three years. This may be due to the standardization of working methods, to 'good housekeeping' measures (of which the separation of the handling of glass-fibre materials from handling the resin mixture may be of utmost importance) and to the development of a nontouch technique (as far as possible). However, in recent investigations Malten (1962) again observed 5 workers sensitized to unsaturated polyester resins: one monovalent, but the others combined and supposingly initiated by sensitizations for epoxy resin ingredients (see Chapter 9, Table 5). From both the Tables 1 and 5 it can be seen, moreover, that group sensitization to unsaturated polyester resins may occur but to a relatively low degree. Laminac 4128, Palatal KR 1144, Palatal P6 were not yet in use at the moment of investigation. The fact that these polyester resins showed scarcely any group-sensitization reactions may be hopeful, although it must be remembered that this does not mean that these compounds may display a smaller sensitization capacity when in actual use. Moreover, it can be read from both tables that sensitizations to the accelerator and the peroxides do occur, but in our experience they are becoming less important as primary sensitizers. This is in contradiction to Wilson *et al.* (1960) who rarely found unsaturated polyester sensitizations, but suspected organic peroxides of having such effect. According to Vale (1953) and Müller (1954) styrene, vinylacetate (see p. 144), butyl and methyl methacrylate (see p. 158), acrylonitrile (see p. 163), may cause dermatitis. According to Schwartz, 1945, and *Hygienic Guide*, 1957, diallyl phthalate (see p. 75), triallyl cyanurate (see p. 75) etc. may be used as cross-linking agents.

Styrene defats the skin, and may give rise to a primary irritation (Hess 1959, Stephenson *et al.* 1960). Sensitizations occur very sporadically if ever in our experience; we only saw one positive patch test in 1956. We, therefore, do not agree with Lieber (1955), who classified it as an outspoken sensitizer. Barsotti *et al.* (1952) reported about two cases of dermatitis pruriginosa in manufacturing polystyrene; confirmation by allergic tests was not reported. It is customary to add *p-tert.*-butyl catechol to prevent spontaneous polymerization of styrene. In former years, this has already been described as an irritant and sensitizer, but Malten (1956) did not find positive patch tests to this substance in persons handling styrene, apparently because of the low concentration in which it is used (10 p.p.m. usually). However, Kendrick (1958) and other authors have found it to be the sensitizer occurring in 'Thermofax' copying paper, in which it may be contained in higher concentration.

From the foregoing it seems that neither the glycols nor the acid anhydride components used to make polyester resins can be accused of causing sensitizations, with the probable exception of fumaric acid. However, one may suspect the esters of phthalic acid and maleic acid. Baader (1955) reported eczema due to diamyl and diethyl phthalate and in our own experience dibutyl maleinate has to be considered as a strong primary skin sensitizer. In an attempt to ascertain the correct patch-testing concentration, 4 out of 6 volunteers became sensitized after one patch test (*cf.* Chapter 6, p. 66). Moreover, a laboratory worker engaged in the synthesis of a semi-stearate of maleic acid became sensitized and showed an exanthema on the ninth day of her work (Mali *et al.* 1961).

SPECIFIC PREVENTION

Stephenson *et al.* (1960) recommended the use of gloves and aprons made of neoprene in working up isopolyesters. Also polyethylene gloves may be used. They advise the use of barrier creams (Ply No. 9, Fend E).

One of the most effective measures in our opinion is to separate the cutting of fibre-glass cloth in the shape wanted and the sanding, drilling and sawing of the cured product from the actual rolling and brushing of the uncured resin in laminating the fibre-glass cloth on moulds, etc. In this way, primary irritation from glass spicules and dust originating from this sort of work (notwithstanding local exhaust ventilation) is obviated in those handling chemicals in their sensitizing phase.

References p. 82

REFERENCES

American Conference Governmental Industrial Hygienists, *Threshold Limit Values*. Detroit, Michigan, 1962.

BAADER, E. W., Erkrankungen durch Phthalsäure und ihre Verbindungen. *Arch. Gewerbepathol. Gewerbehyg.*, 13 (1955) 419.

BARDODEJ, Z., B. MALEK, B. VOLFOVA and E. ZELENA, Dangers in the use of styrene in the manufacture of plastic/glass laminates. *Czech. Hyg.*, 5 (1960) 541. Ref.: *C.I.S. Docum., Dafi Xkz Gfz.*, 238, 1961.

BARSOTTI, M., L. PARMEGGIANI and C. SASSI, Observations on occupational pathology in a polystyrene resin factory. *Med. Lavoro*, 43 (1952) 418. Ref.: *Arch. Ind. Hyg.*, 7 (1953) 358.

BROWNING, E., *Toxicity of industrial organic solvents*. H.M.S.O., London, 1953.

BROWNING, E., Toxic solvents: a review. *Brit. J. Ind. Med.*, 16 (1959) 23.

Chemical Safety Data Sheet SD-37, *Styrene Monomer*. Manufact. Chemists' Assoc., Washington, 1951.

DROGICINA, E. A., G. N. MAZUNINA, A. A. ORLOWA, H. M. RASCHEWSKAJA and E. A. SOLOWIEWA, Klinik der chronischen Vergiftung bei der Herstellung von synthetischen Divinylsterol und Chloropreen Kautschuk. *Gigiena Truda i Prof. Zabolevaniya*, 3 (1959) 10. Ref.: *Zbl. Arbeitsmed.*, 11 (1961) 199.

DUNLAP, M. K., J. K. KODAMA, J. S. WELLINGTON, H. H. ANDERSON and C. H. HINE, The toxicity of allyl alcohol. *Arch. Ind. Health*, 18 (1958) 303.

EICH, J., Arbeitssicherheit beim Umgang mit zweikomponenten Kunststoffen. *Zbl. Arbeitsmed.*, 10 (1960) 205.

FEUER, S. S., T. E. BOCKSTAHLER, C. A. BROWN and I. ROSENTHAL, Maleic–fumaric isomerization in unsaturated polyesters. *Ind. Eng. Chem.*, 46 (1954) 1643.

HAGEN, U., *Glasfaser verstärkte Kunststoffe*, Springer, Berlin, 1956.

HARTOGENSIS, F., Onderzoek in een afdeling voor gewapende kunststoffen; industrieel-hygiënische aspecten. *Tijdschr. Soc. Geneesk.*, 40 (1962) 223.

HESS, W., Schutzmassnahmen bei der Verarbeitung von Niederdruckharzen. *Schweiz. Bl. Arb. Sicherheit*, 22, juli 1959.

HOFMANN, H. T., Zur Frage der Gesundheitsgefährdung durch moderne Kunststoffe und ihre Lösungsmittel. *Zbl. Arbeitsmed.*, 11 (1961) 240.

HOWELL, J., Contact dermatitis. *Arch. Dermatol. Syphilol. (Chicago)*, 53 (1946) 265.

Hygienic Guide, Acrylonitrile. *Am. Ind. Hyg. Assoc. Quart.*, 18 (1957) 78.

JONGH, J., Onderzoek in een afdeling voor gewapende kunststoffen; bedrijfsgeneeskundige aspecten. *Tijdschr. Soc. Geneesk.*, 40 (1962) 219.

KALSBEEK, J. W. H., and R. L. ZIELHUIS, Unpublished investigations about styrene, Leiden, 1960.

KENDRICK, F. J., Dermatitis caused by a copying paper. *Arch. Dermatol.*, 77 (1958) 334.

KLAUDER, J. V., Sensitization dermatitis from 'Scottissue' towels. *Arch. Dermatol. Syphilol. (Chicago)*, 57 (1948) 414.

KLIMKOVA-DEUTSCHOVA, E., Neurologische Befunde in der Plastikindustrie bei Styrol Arbeitern. *Int. Arch. Gewerbepathol. Gewerbehyg.*, 19 (1962) 35.

LIEBER, E. E., Dermatitis – an industrial problem. *Brit. Plastics*, 28 (1955) 428.

LOESER, A., and G. BORNEMANN, Biologische Wirkungen von monomeren Styrol. *Fette, Seifen, Anstrichmittel*, 58 (1956) 181.

MALI, J. W. H., K. E. MALTEN and F. C. J. VAN NEER, Etiologie en pathogenese van de margarine-ziekte. *Ned. Tijdschr. Geneesk.*, 105 (1961) 801.

MALTEN, K. E., *Beroepsekseem bij het verwerken van kunststoffen.* Thesis, Amsterdam, 1956.

MALTEN, K. E., Unpublished investigation, Nijmegen, 1962.

MÜLLER, A., Chemie der ungesättigten Polyesterharze bei ihrer Herstellung und Verarbeitung. *Kunststoffe*, 44 (1954) 578.

POKROWSKY, W. A., On the toxicity of styrol. *Gigiena Truda i Prof. Zabolevaniya*, 5 (1961) No. 5, p. 3.

ROGERS, J. C., Industrial hygiene problems in the field of plastics. *Arch. Ind. Health*, 12 (1955) 470.

ROWE, V. K., G. J. ATCHINSON, E. N. LUCE and E. M. ADAMS, The determination of monomeric styrene in air. *J. Ind. Hyg.*, 25 (1943) 348.

RYLOVA, M. L., Toxic action of styrene and α-methylstyrene. *Gigiena i Sanit.*, 5 (1955) 21. Ref.: KLIMKOVA, 1962.

SCHWARTZ, L., Skin hazards in the manufacture and processing of synthetic rubber. *J. Am. Med. Assoc.*, 127 (1945) 389.

SPECTOR, W. S., *Handbook of Toxicology*, Vol. I, Saunders, Philadelphia, 1956.

SPENCER, H. C., D. D. IRISH, E. M. ADAMS and V. K. ROWE, Response of laboratory animals to monomeric styrene. *J. Ind. Hyg.*, 24 (1942) 295.

STEPHENSON, R. W. and L. B. FOSDICK, Hazards in the use of polyesters as maintenance coatings. *Am. Ind. Hyg. Assoc. J.*, 21 (1960) 522.

TORKELSON, T. R., M. A. WOLF, F. OYEN and V. K. ROWE, Vapor toxicity of allyl chloride as determined on laboratory animals. *Am. Ind. Hyg. Assoc. J.*, 20 (1959a) 217.

TORKELSON, T. R., M. A. WOLF, F. OYEN and V. K. ROWE, Vapor toxicity of allyl alcohol as determined on laboratory animals. *Am. Ind. Hyg. Assoc. J.*, 20 (1959b) 224.

TUCHENKO, M. M. and P. V. BIDYAKOW, Issues of industrial hygiene in the production of glass plastics. *Gigiena Truda i prof. Zabolevaniya*, 5 (1961) 20.

VALE, C. P., The chemistry of unsaturated polyester resins. *Brit. Plastics*, 24 (1953) 327.

WILSON, R. H. and W. E. MCCORMICK, Plastics. *Arch. Ind. Health*, 21 (1960) 536.

WINSEMIUS, W., Onderzoek in een afdeling voor gewapende kunststoffen; psychologische aspecten. *Tijdschr. Soc. Geneesk.*, 40 (1962) 229.

WOLF, M. A., V. K. ROWE, D. D. MCCOLLISTER, R. L. HOLLINGSWORTH and F. OYEN, Toxicological studies of certain alkylated benzenes and benzene. *Arch. Ind. Health*, 14 (1956) 387.

ZAWADZKI, S., A rapid method for detecting styrene in the atmosphere. *Prace Centr. Inst. Ochrony Pracy (Warsaw)*, 11 (1961) 27. Ref.: *C.I.S. Docum., Dafi Qix*, 1770–1961.

ZIELHUIS, R. L., Medisch-hygienische aspecten van de verwerking van gewapende kunststoffen. *Veiligheid*, 38 (1962a) 25.

ZIELHUIS, R. L., De relatie tussen expositie aan oplosmiddelen en verschijnselen van intoxicatie. *Tijdschr. Soc. Geneesk.*, 40 (1962b) 225.

8

Isocyanates

PHYSICO-CHEMICAL PROPERTIES, APPLICATION

Isocyanates are compounds with isocyanate groups (–N=C=O). If they possess at least two such groups, they may take part in the production of high-polymer compounds: the nitrogen atom accepts a reactive hydrogen atom from a different type of monomer, linking the carbon atom of the isocyanate group with the activated group of that other monomer (polyaddition–polymerization); linkage therefore does not occur between two C-atoms as in most other polymers, but between hetero-atoms.

Generally, isocyanates are able to react with all compounds bearing groups which possess a hydrogen atom replaceable by sodium: –OH, –COOH, $-NH_2$, $-SO_2NH_2$. *In vivo*, for instance, they link very well with proteins.

In industry, tridimensional high-molecular products are mostly produced by the reaction of di-isocyanates with polyhydroxy compounds. These products are called *polyurethanes.*

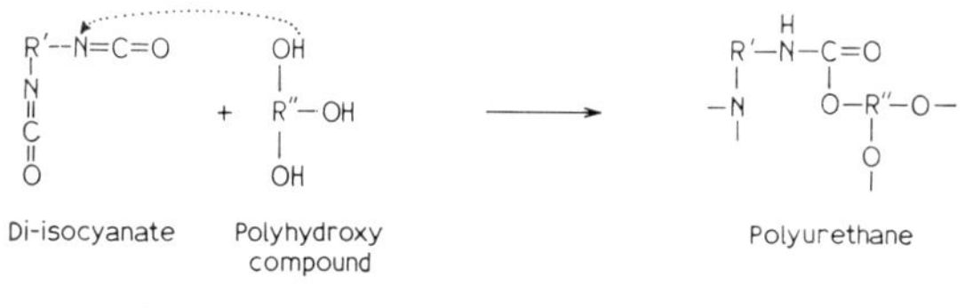

In industry, the isocyanate component and the polyhydroxy component are generally added together shortly before proces-

References p. 98

sing. This, therefore, takes place with an incompletely cured mixture. Thus curing occurs during the moulding process.

Methods for determination of isocyanate concentration in the industrial atmosphere have been presented by Ehrlicher (1956), Zapp (1957), Marcali (1959), I.C.I. (1959) and Robinson (1962).

Decomposition of polymers occurs at 220–275° (Strayer 1959); isocyanates and N-oxides are produced. Decomposition experiments with Moltopren(TDI), Vulkollan(NDI) and rigid foam(MDI) at temperatures from 300–1000° did not yield any free monomers, but only small amounts of HCN, CO, low-molecular polyurethanes, toluene diamine (Ehrlicher 1962).

Applications

Polyurethane lacquers

Polyesters with free OH-groups (often called Desmophens) are linked with di-isocyanates (called Desmodurs). Because of the rather short pot-life it is necessary to apply the two-component mixture immediately after mixing. The curing takes place partly *after* the spraying or brushing has been done. As solvents and thinners, esters, ketones, chlorinated and aromatic hydrocarbons are used. Because of the serious hygienic aspects (see p. 92) of the originally applied very volatile compounds, hexamethylene di-isocyanate and toluylene di-isocyanate have been abandoned for the greater part. Nowadays less volatile and much less hazardous compounds such as Desmodur L or diphenylmethane–di-isocyanate are used.

Artificial fibres

Linear polymers built from glycols and di-isocyanates.

Polyurethane foam plastic

From a hygienic point of view (see below) a distinction should be made between *flexible* foams, based upon a reaction between polyesters or polyethers and toluylene di-isocyanate and *rigid* foams, because the latter nowadays are based upon less-volatile compounds (such as diphenylmethane–di-isocyanate). Triethylene diamine and alkaline phenolates are used as catalysts. As foaming agents, freons may be used. It is also possible to add a surplus of isocyanates and H_2O which produces CO_2 as foaming agent.

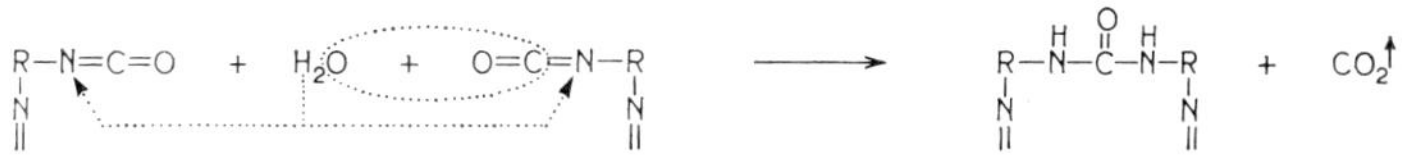

Because this reaction is exotherm, the risk of evaporation of more or less volatile monomers is rather large; moreover, the produced CO_2 will carry isocyanates into the atmosphere (Zapp 1957; Walworth *et al.* 1959). Unreacted monomers may be set free by rolling polyether foams (in order to open the closed foam cells). If too great a surplus of isocyanates is added, the internal temperature may rise to 400–500°; in that case there is a serious risk of spontaneous combustion and emanation of monomers (Knop 1960, 1961).

Foam plastics may be produced *in situ* by spraying the two components separately by means of a dual spray gun.

Rubbers

Linear polyesters are linked with di-isocyanates, for instance glycol–adipic acid esters with 1,5-naphthalene di-isocyanate; H_2O, dialcohols, diamines and other bifunctional compounds are used as catalysts.

Glue

e.g. tri-isocyanate–triphenylmethane. Polyisocyanate glues are used for instance to glue rubber on textiles, metals or ceramic articles.

As many isocyanates are principally known under trade names, the most important of these may be enumerated (Table 2).

The boiling points and vapour pressures (volatility) of the compounds may differ considerably; Hampton *et al.* (1960) presented the examples given in Table 3.

References p. 98

TABLE 2

TRADE NAMES OF ISOCYANATES

Desmodur H	=	hexamethylene di-isocyanate.
Desmodur HH	=	condensation product of Desmodur H and trimethylol propane.
Desmodur O	=	trimer of Desmodur H.
Desmodur T	=	TDI = 2,4- and 2,6-toluene diisocyanate = Suprasec E, EN, SF, SFN.
Desmodur TT	=	dimer of Desmodur T (activated at 150°).
Desmodur TH	=	condensation product of Desmodur T and a triol; contains about 10% Desmodur T.
Desmodur THN	=	condensation product of Desmodur T; contains a small % of Desmodur T.
Desmodur L	=	idem, contains less than 0.5% Desmodur T.
Desmodur AP	=	Desmodur TH + phenol; TDI is set free at 150°.
Desmodur R	=	4,4,4-tri-isocyanato–triphenylmethane.
NDI	=	1,5-naphthylene di-isocyanate.
MDI	=	Suprasec D (A) = 4,4-di-isocyanato-diphenylmethane = Desmodur 44 V.
p-PDI	=	*p*-phenylene di-isocyanate.
XDI	=	4,4-xenylene di-isocyanate.

The factors which determine air pollution by isocyanates especially in regard to paint application were studied by Ehrlicher (1956), Funke *et al.* (1958) and Hampton *et al.* (1960).

TABLE 3

BOILING POINTS AND VAPOUR PRESSURES OF ISOCYANATES

	b.p. in degrees °C	*v.p. in mm Hg/ 25° C*
Desmodur H	132°/15 mm Hg	1.0×10^{-2}
Desmodur T = TDI	131°/16 mm Hg	2.3×10^{-2}
MDI	215–217°/15 mm Hg	about 10^{-5}
Desmodur R	240°/0.75 mm Hg	undeterminable

The results of their investigations with TDI, Desmodur TH, Desmodur THN, Desmodur L and MDI may be summarized as follows:

a. The concentration in air decreased with smaller percentages of free TDI in the compound; the *volatility* of the isocyanate component is of primary importance.

b. *Spraying* always yielded higher concentrations in air than application by brush; spraying of MDI, however, did not cause concentrations beyond 0.1 p.p.m. in air.

c. The concentration in air decreased with shorter *drying time* (dependent on temperature, humidity, catalyst, type of isocyanate).

d. The concentration in air increased when more volatile *solvents* were used.

Manufacturing of rigid polyurethane *foams*, based upon MDI, even in industrial practice, gave rise to concentrations far below 0.1 p.p.m. (I.C.I. 1959), in sharp contrast with the older methods based upon TDI.

EXPERIMENTAL TOXICOLOGY AND DERMATOLOGY

Subcutaneous injection of even large quantities of TDI in mice (Grosz *et al.* 1941) or guinea pigs (Fuchs *et al.* 1951) did not cause systemic effects. The compound however was irritating for rabbit skin and eye, without any indication of percutaneous resorption. Exposure of dogs, guinea pigs and rabbits to 1000–2000 mg TDI/m^3 was very irritating to the respiratory tract. In accordance with clinical experience from industry, most experimental work has been centered on this phenomenon.

Friebel *et al.* (1955) injected intratracheally 0.3 ml TDI in guinea pigs. The animals died quickly from respiratory distress; coagulation of proteins in the respiratory tract occurred. Exposure of guinea pigs to 1200 mg TDI/m^3 in aerosol or 350–550 mg/m^3 as vapour for 10–20 min at irregular intervals for one month caused asthmatic reactions after the first few inhalations,

References p. 98

changing into continuous dyspnoea in the course of the experiment. Bronchiolitis obliterans, pneumonia and emphysema occurred with a very small tendency to healing. Guinea pigs sensitized to chicken albumen responded in the same manner as non-treated animals. Friebel *et al.* arrived at the conclusion that a primary toxic effect seemed to predominate (no typical response to spasmolytics; attacks occurred after a latency period; respiration curves atypical for sensitization asthma). Allergic components, however, could not be completely excluded.

In experiments reported by Zapp (1957) exposure to 600 p.p.m. TDI (4200 mg/m^3) for 6 h was lethal for rats; 60 p.p.m. did not cause deaths. Repeated exposure of rats, guinea pigs, rabbits or dogs to 1–2 p.p.m. TDI (7–14 mg/m^3) for 0.5–6 h, however, always gave rise to congestion and inflammation of the respiratory tract: bronchitis and sometimes pneumonia; asthmatic attacks were not observed. The oral LD_{50} for rats was high: 5800 mg TDI/kg. The irritating properties to animal skin and eyes were confirmed, even if 10% TDI in dimethyl phthalate was applied. Zapp concluded that TDI had a rather low oral toxicity, but because of the effects of repeated exposure to low concentrations, he proposed a MAC of 0.1 p.p.m. = 0.7 mg/m^3. Henschler *et al.* (1962) exposed rats and guinea pigs repeatedly to 0.1 p.p.m.; they did not observe any clear lung pathology, but the body weight increased less. Duncan *et al.* (1962) established the following 14-day LC_{50}: 13.9 p.p.m. (rats), 12.7 p.p.m. (guinea pigs), 11.0 p.p.m. (rabbits), 9.7 p.p.m. (mice). Intratracheal spraying of NDI also caused bronchiolitis obliterans in rabbits; fibroplasia occurred in the bronchial lumen, but hardly in the interstitial tissue itself (Klavis *et al.* 1959). Carcinogenic properties were not observed (Williams 1959).

Pyrolysis of polyurethane foam at 200–560° yielded toxic products: exposed rats died from pulmonary edema; pyrolysis products of neoprene, latex or PVC, however, possessed the same order of toxicity (Zapp 1957). McFarland *et al.* (1962)

determined the toxicity of pyrolysis products of polyurethane foam (A), or nylon coated with this foam (B). The pyrolysis products were much more toxic in rats. At a given concentration, the pyrolysis products of A killed faster than the products of B, but the proportion of animals ultimately dying was smaller. A-products caused acute asphyxia by bronchiolar occlusion; B-products caused pulmonary edema. The authors warned against the danger of fire of polyurethane-coated clothes.

Ehrlicher *et al.* (1956) exposed human subjects for 1 min to an aerosol of TDI. They noted a slight aromatic odour at 0.13 p.p.m., a definite odour without irritation at 0.60 p.p.m., a burning feeling in eyes and nose at 1.9 p.p.m. and a severe irritation of eyes and respiratory tract at 3.9 p.p.m. The odour threshold was also determined by Strayer (1959); 50% of 24 subjects had a minimum threshold of 0.4 p.p.m. (vapour); irritation occurred at 0.5 p.p.m. Also Munn (1960) observed lower values for irritation than Ehrlicher *et al.*: 0.1 to 0.2 p.p.m. (vapour) caused a definite odour, concentrations above 0.2 p.p.m. were definitely irritating. According to Henschler *et al.* (1962) the odour threshold was even 0.05 p.p.m. TDI. The odour of isocyanates is not a valuable warning signal, because the MAC value is much lower (0.02 p.p.m., see p. 97) and because, particularly in paint application, the odour of solvents provides a masking effect.

Tests on guinea pig skin confirmed the local irritant action of TDI even when applied to intact skin as a 10% solution in dimethyl phthalate. In addition it was possible to produce allergic skin sensitization of guinea pigs with TDI (Zapp 1957). By means of a prophetic patch test with polyurethane-foam plastic in more than 200 subjects Zapp (1957) did not observe any sensitization and hardly any irritation, although the cured polyurethane foams might be presumed still to contain a number of free isocyanate groups (Tolot *et al.* 1961), if for some reason they had escaped reaction with water or moisture in the air.

INDUSTRIAL TOXICOLOGY AND DERMATOLOGY

Industrial exposure to isocyanates mainly results in a rather uniform pattern of reaction: irritation of the respiratory tract. After exposure to hazardous concentrations more or less severe signs of irritation of the air passages occur, manifesting itself in 'asthmatic bronchitis' over a range of slight difficulty in breathing to severe asthmatic state. The period of previous exposure may be a few hours, but also days, weeks or months. Prodromal signs (irritation of upper air passages, 'cold') may precede more definite ones. Severe complaints generally occur some hours after the exposure has ended. The intensity is determined by concentration in air, duration of exposure and individual predisposition. Subjects with a negative history of respiratory tract disorders, however, are certainly not 'immune' to the agent. More frequently than an acute asthmatic attack, a subacute syndrome of pulmonary oppression with severe coughing fits (particularly at night, causing sleeplessness) and dyspnoea ensues. Bronchospasm is present; the ventilatory function is decreased. Signs of systemic toxicity rarely occur; they may be due to other toxic agents, *e.g.* solvents. A moderate eosinophilia (below 10%) is sometimes found; it should not be regarded as diagnostic. If the exposure does not continue, relief of symptoms generally occurs within a few days to weeks, accompanied by an amelioration of lung function. In some cases, however, relief is not achieved, a chronic obliterating bronchitis develops; at last the patient may develop fatal cor pulmonale. The irritation of the respiratory tract therefore may result in death, either in an acute asthmatic state, or after a long period of disability. If relief of symptoms occurs, an increased susceptibility (allergy or hyper-reactive mucosa) is apt to follow.

In two workers, Rutgers (1962) established a reversible unequal ventilation, disturbed ventilation–perfusion ratio, and hypotonia of the bronchus wall. In one case, in addition to a progressive disability lasting for 6 years, due to asthmatic bronchitis and bronchiectasis (after exposure for only 2 days (!) to TDI and Desmodur THN), Leupold (1960) also observed a flaccid paralysis of the legs; whether or not this was related to the original intoxication was not clear. Nakanishi *et al.* (1958) described 18 cases in an exposed group of 54 workers; some of them also showed dermatitis, gastric disorders and anorexia (the data are not complete enough to exclude other possible agents). Baader (1956) once found on autopsy a small cellular reticulosis. Jennings *et al.* (1963) observed thrombocytopenic purpura in two cases.

The dermatological hazard seems to be very small. Local application in the eyes may cause severe conjunctivitis.

Since the publication of Fuchs *et al.* (1951) many authors have recorded their experiences from industry, offering a rather depressing, monotonous series of signs of irritation of the respiratory tract. Some isocyanates certainly may be regarded as very hazardous monomers.

Fuchs *et al.* (1951) observed the syndrome in 7 of 9 subjects, exposed for less than 2 months to TDI, applied in a plastifier for vinyl resins; some complaints of asthenia and gastric disorders may have been due to simultaneous exposure to other agents, *e.g.* azoisobutyronitrile (see p. 223).

The application of two-component polyurethane lacquers containing TDI has been an important source of cases up to 1959. Reinl (1953) described the first accidents from this category; one of the patients died after a disability of 8 years, another developed a high degree of susceptibility. Two fatalities, either in an asthmatic state (accompanied by urticaria) or after an invalidism of 6 years were reported by Schürmann (1955). One painter developed a fatal asthma after an exposure of only 5 days (Gerritsen 1955). Swensson *et al.* (1955) and Bosshard (1959) recorded two series of cases. Bosshard observed 81 non-severe cases in painters; 93 % of them were dyspnoeic, 80 % showed signs of tracheitis or asthmatic bronchitis; relief always occurred within 3 weeks; in 32 subjects the exposure only lasted for one day. Schur (1959) also observed symptoms within one

References p. 98

day of exposure; one of the subjects still had a decreased lung function after 9 months. Since 1959, however, cases from this field have not been reported any longer; this is undoubtedly mainly due to replacement of TDI by the much less hazardous newer isocyanates MDI or Desmodur L. Care should still be taken to protect against inhalation of tiny droplets of these relatively non-volatile compounds. Baader (1960) and Seidel *et al.* (1960) still described cases due to application of lacquers based on 'masked' isocyanates (Desmodur AP releases TDI at 150°); in 4 female workers asthmatic bronchitis occurred after coating Desmodur AP-enamelled wire with tin for 4 weeks.

A very important source of sometimes very serious intoxications has been and still is the production of polyurethane foam plastics, based also upon TDI. In Germany cases were reported by Reinl (1953), Ganz *et al.* (1954) and Schürmann (1955) from the production of Moltopren; in some cases exposure only lasted one day. Ehrlicher *et al.* (1956) did not observe any complaints in workers when exposed to an average concentration of 0.16 p.p.m. TDI (with a long-lasting increase to 0.3 p.p.m.) in the production of foam plastics. In a group of 25 workers, observed by Woodbury (1956) for 1.5 year, 8 subjects had signs of bronchospasm; individual predisposition was evident. Examination of internal organs (liver, kidney, blood) did not reveal any pathology. Johnstone (1957) and Johnstone *et al.* (1960) reported 17 and 23 cases of asthmatic bronchitis due to TDI in the production of foam plastics; 4 workers became ill after an exposure as short as 1 to 5 days. Neither X-ray examination nor investigation of liver and blood revealed any pathology. According to Hama (1957) exposure to 0.03–0.07 p.p.m. TDI resulted in slight to severe 'colds', which disappeared when the exposure decreased to 0.01–0.03 p.p.m. Similar experiences were reported by Sands *et al.* (1957): 42 cases of intoxication (9 of them serious) occurred at exposures beyond 0.1 p.p.m. TDI new cases did not arise at exposures to 0.04–0.06 p.p.m. (average). Walworth *et al.* (1959) observed 83 cases of intoxication after

3 to 4 weeks exposure to 0.17 p.p.m. TDI (average per month; max. 2.2 p.p.m.); when the monthly average decreased to 0.01–0.1 p.p.m. the number of new cases was much less, but recurrence of symptoms still occurred in previously diseased persons even at these low concentrations. The above-mentioned experiences from American industries are definitely more unfavourable than the data of Ehrlicher *et al.* (1956) mentioned above. Kessler (1960) reported symptoms in a worker, mixing TDI 4 times for about 5 minutes in the course of 2.5 months; after the 3rd exposure moderate irritation, after the 4th exposure acute asthma occurred. Trenchard *et al.* (1963) described an 'epidemic' of respiratory symptoms due to TDI in a factory producing foams. At least 12 cases were diagnosed; at first all of them were thought to suffer from 'influenza'. These workers themselves were not working with the product, but in a department 'downwind' in the ventilation system, whereas the directly exposed workers were effectively wearing respiratory protective apparatus.

From the hygienic viewpoint the rigid foams should be distinguished from the flexible foams. In the production of the former the technical development made the application possible of the much less hazardous MDI. Munn (1960), who observed several cases of intoxication from exposure to TDI did not see any disturbances of health while exposed to MDI. Experiences of Williams (1959), I.C.I. (1959), Walpole *et al.* (1959), Hampton *et al.* (1960) also proved that production of rigid foams *in situ* was non-hazardous. Only Johnstone *et al.* (1960) mentioned one case of intoxication after exposure to MDI (in monochlorobenzene). The data of Munn (1960) perhaps may explain this exception: at the beginning he also observed 'MDI' intoxications, but at that moment MDI proved to contain 10% TDI; the newer types of MDI contain only negligible amounts of TDI. According to Ehrlicher (1962) the older types of Desmodur 44V contained phenyl isocyanate as an irritant impurity.

Exposure to naphthylene di-isocyanate and *m*-phenylene di-

References p. 98

isocyanate has also been reported as a cause of intoxication (Goldblatt 1956; Seidel *et al.* 1960).

In only one instance exposure to the cured polyurethane foam plastic itself has resulted in allergic symptoms (Tolot *et al.*, 1961): a female supervisor in a toy factory developed subsequently conjunctivitis, stomatitis and pharyngitis, and a slight asthmatic reaction; skin tests were positive for the foam plastic. Other workers in the same department did not reveal any symptoms.

Another problem is the thermal decomposition of the plastic: Bergtholdt (1961) reported symptoms in 21 workers cutting foam-covered steel at a naval ship yard. Rutgers (1962) observed severe intoxications in workers exposed to fumes from welding a TDI pump.

It is still a disputed question whether the clinical signs are due to primary irritation or to allergy. A few cases certainly seem to point to an allergic state: a recurrence of asthmatic reaction is caused by minimal contact with the offending agent. Presumably, most cases are due to primary toxic effects: clinical symptoms may arise already after exposure for some hours or a few days (no period of development of hypersensitivity); the asthmatic reaction mostly occurs after exposure has ended (as in phosgene intoxication); the data from animal experiments also point to a primary toxic effect. The presence of a moderate eosinophilia certainly does not prove allergy. Apparently, Goldblatt (1956) was not right to regard aliphatic isocyanates as primary toxic agents and aromatic isocyanates as allergens; the industrial experiences recorded do not confirm this hypothesis.

Seidel *et al.* (1960) summarized the different possible pathogenic mechanisms as follows:

- primary toxic damage by the isocyanates themselves;
- allergy to decomposition of mucosa proteins;
- allergy to bacteria, multiplying in the damaged mucosa;
- allergy to solvents, plastifiers, etc.;
- allergy to the isocyanates themselves.

The first mentioned hypothesis is probably the most valid. In the introduction to this chapter the binding capacity of isocyanates to proteins is mentioned, thus one would anticipate the formation of a complete antigen-compound in consequence of which sensitizations might occur. However, according to Zapp (1957), contact eczema is rare among workers preparing polymers based on the isocyanates. This may be partly due to the fact that due to the irritating nature of the material, it is naturally handled with caution. Reports on urticaria due to use of two-component polyurethane lacquers (Schürmann 1955) remain scarce. In regard to the allergy hypothesis, however, the recent observations reported by Stokinger (1962) should be mentioned: rabbits inhaling low levels of TDI (0.1 p.p.m.) repeatedly showed the development of potent agglutinins.

SPECIFIC PREVENTION

Intoxication by isocyanates is caused exclusively by inhalation. Primary toxic effects preponderate. Decrease of the isocyanate concentration in air is therefore the most valid preventive measure. Zapp (1957) proposed a MAC of 0.1 p.p.m., which, at first, was generally accepted. More recent observations however threw doubt upon the acceptability of this value. In 1961 the American Conference of Governmental Industrial Hygienists therefore proposed a much lower value of 0.02 p.p.m. = 0.14 mg/m^3 for toluylene di-isocyanate; according to this authority even this value does not always protect against recurrence of symptoms after renewed exposure. Elkins *et al.* (1962) consider 0.01 p.p.m. as a reasonable limit for unprotected workers.

The producer firms, acknowledging the serious implications of the di-isocyanates, succeeded in making new products, which are much less hazardous, because less volatile. The newer isocyanates nowadays are generally applied in paints and rigid foams, but the production of flexible foams still has to make use

References p. 98

of the older, more volatile products. Specific prevention measures for workers spraying foam upon tank surfaces were given by Peterson *et al.* (1962).

Extensive safety measures are given by *Chemical Safety Data-Sheet* SD-73 (1959). The very strict regulations, formerly set for application of polyurethane paints, could be mitigated in recent years. If the new isocyanates are applied, the hazard corresponds to the hazard of cellulose paints.

First-aid measures are extensively described in the Data Sheet mentioned above. The skin should not be cleansed with acetone, but with cellosolve followed by washing with much water and soap (Walpole *et al.* 1959; Williams 1959). Eyes should be rinsed copiously with water at once. Spilt isocyanates should be absorbed by a special powder.

In pre-employment examination, special attention should be paid to the respiratory tract.

REFERENCES

American Conference Governmental Industrial Hygienists, *Threshold Limit Values*, Detroit, Michigan, 1961.

BAADER, E. W., *Arbeitsmedizin in Europa*, Steinkopf, Darmstadt, 1956.

BAADER, E. W., *Klinische Grundlagen der sechsundvierzig meldepflichtigen Berufskrankheiten*, Urban & Schwarzenberg, Munich, 1960.

BERGTHOLDT, C. P. I., Recent welding practice at naval facilities. *Arch. Environ. Health*, 2 (1961) 257.

BOSSHARD, R., Gewerbemedizinische Aspekte der beruflichen Gefahren im Malergewerbe. *Z. Unfallmed. Berufskr.*, 52 (1959) 218.

Chemical Safety Data Sheet, SD-73. *Toluylene diisocyanate*, Manufact. Chemists' Assoc., Washington, 1959.

DUNCAN, B., L. D. SCHEEL, E. J. FAIRCHILD, R. KILLANS and S. GRAHAM, Toluene diisocyanate inhalation toxicity, pathology and mortality. *Am. Ind. Hyg. Assoc. J.*, 23 (1962) 447.

EHRLICHER, H., Zur Frage der Arbeitsplatzüberwachung in Toluylen-diisocyanate herstellenden und verarbeitenden Betrieben. *Zbl. Arbeitsmed.*, 6 (1956) 138.

EHRLICHER, H., Arbeitsmedizinische Fragen auf dem Kunststoff-gebiet. *Kongress für Arbeitsschutz 1961*, Steinkopf, Darmstadt, 1962.

EHRLICHER, H. and W. PILZ, Industriehygienische und Arbeitsmedizinische Massnahmen bei der Verwendung von Isocyanaten (Desmodur) und die analytische Bestimmung einiger aromatischer Isocyanate. *Arbeitsschutz*, 1956, p. 276 and 1957, p. 7.

ELKINS, H. B., G. W. MCCARL and H. G. BRUGSCH, Massachusetts experience with toluene diisocyanate. *Am. Ind. Hyg. Assoc. J.*, 23 (1962) 265.

FRIEBEL, H. and H. LÜCHTRATH, Zur Wirkung von Toluylendiisocyanat (Desmodur). *Naunyn-Schmiedeberg's Arch. exptl. Pathol. Pharmakol.*, 227 (1955) 93.

FUCHS, S. and P. VALADE, Étude clinique et expérimentale sur quelques cas d'intoxication par le Desmodur T. *Arch. Maladies Prof.*, 12 (1951) 191.

FUNKE, W. and K. HAMANN, Die Bestimmung von flüchtigem Isocyanat bei Desmophen–Desmodur-Anstrichen. *Farbe und Lack*, 64 (1958) 120.

GANZ, H. and E. MAGER, Gesundheitsschäden durch den Schaumstoff Moltopren. *Zbl. Arbeitsmed.*, 4 (1954) 42.

GERRITSEN, W. B., Asthma door beroepsinvloeden, i.h.b. door isocyanaten. *Chem. Weekblad*, 51 (1955) 269.

GOLDBLATT, M. W., in E. R. A. MEREWETHER (Ed.), *Industrial Medicine and Hygiene*, Vol. III, Butterworth, London, 1956.

GROSZ and HELLRUNG, Unpublished investigations, 1941. Ref.: REINL, 1953.

HAMA, G. M., Symptoms in workers exposed to isocyanates. *Arch. Ind. Health*, 16 (1957) 232.

HAMPTON, H. A., R. HURD and H. J. SHEARING, Recent developments in polyurethanes. *J. Oil & Colour Chemists' Assoc.*, 43 (1960) 96.

HENSCHLER, D., W. ASSMANN and K. O. MEYER, Zur Toxikologie der Toluylenediisocyanate. *Arch. Toxikol.*, 19 (1962) 364.

Hygienic Guide. Toluene 2,4-diisocyanate. *Am. Ind. Hyg. Assoc. Quart.*, 18 (1957) 370.

Imperial Chemical Industries, Urethane. *Technical information*, PC/U. 11 (1959).

JENNINGS, G. H. and N. D. GOWER, Thrombocytopenic purpura in toluene diisocyanate workers. *Lancet*, *i* (1963) 406.

JOHNSTONE, R. T., Toluene 2,4-diisocyanate. *Ind. Med. Surg.*, 26 (1957) 33.

JOHNSTONE, R. T. and S. E. MILLER, *Occupational Diseases and Industrial Medicine*, Saunders, Philadelphia, 1960.

KESSLER, R. C., Pulmonary sensitization to toluene diisocyanate. *J. Occupational Med.*, 2 (1960) 143.

KLAVIS, G. and L. C. SCHULZ, Tierexperimentelle Untersuchungen über spezifische Wirkungen und Spätfolgen nach Desmodur 15. *Arch. Toxikol.*, 17 (1959) 338.

KNOP, W., Selbstentzündung von Schaumstoffabfällen. *Zbl. Arbeitsmed.*, 10 (1960) 216.

KNOP, W., Nochmals Selbstenzündung von Schaumstoffabfällen. *Zbl. Arbeitsmed.*, 11 (1961) 250.

LEUPOLD, F., Beitrag zur Frage der Schädigung durch Isocyanate. *Ärztl. Wochschr.*, 15 (1960) 74.

McFARLAND, H. N. and K. J. LEONG, Hazards from the thermodecomposition of plastics. *Arch. Environ. Health*, 4 (1962) 591.

MARCALI, K., Microdetermination of toluene diisocyanates in atmosphere. *Arch. Ind. Health*, 19 (1959) 354.

MUNN, A., Experiences with diisocyanates. *Trans. Assoc. Ind. Med. Officers*, 9 (1960) 134.

NAKANISHI, S. and S. NAMIKI, Erscheinungen bei isocyanatgefährdeten Arbeitern. *Rodo Kagaku*, 34 (1958) 980. Ref.: *Zbl. Arbeitsmed.*, 10 (1960) 118.

PETERSON, J. A., R. A. COPELAND and H. R. HOYLE, Health hazards of spraying polyurethane foams. *Am. Ind. Hyg. Assoc. J.*, 23 (1962) 345.

REINL, W., Über Erkrankungen bei der Verarbeitung von Kunststoffen auf der Basis der Polyurethane. *Zbl. Arbeitsmed.*, 3 (1953) 103.

ROBINSON, D. R., Atmospheric determination of toluylene diisocyanate. *Am. Ind. Hyg. Assoc. J.*, 23 (1962) 228.

RUTGERS, V. H., Waarnemingen bij arbeiders blootgesteld aan 2,4-tolueen diisocyanaat (Desmodur T). *Ned. Tijdschr. Geneesk.*, 106, II (1962) 1726.

SANDS, F. W., G. BOFFARDI and K. E. JAMES, Toluene diisocyanate. *Am. Ind. Hyg. Assoc. Quart.*, 18 (1957) 331.

SCHÜRMANN, D., Gesundheitsschäden durch neuartige Lacke und Schaumstoffe. *Deut. Med. Wochschr.*, 80 (1955) 1661.

SCHUR, E., Schädigung durch Desmodur Lacke; Reizgas oder Allergie? *Med. Klin. (München)*, 54 (1959) 168.

SEIDEL, H. and H. POHLE, Zur Schädigung der Atmungsorgane durch Desmodure. *Tuberkulosearzt*, 14 (1960) 675.

STOKINGER, H. E., New concepts and future trends in toxicology. *Am. Industr. Hyg. Assoc. J.*, 23 (1962) 8.

STRAYER, I. C., Safe use and safe handling of organic isocyanates. *Arch. Ind. Health*, 19 (1959) 351.

SWENSSON, A., E. HOLMQVIST and K. D. LUNDGREN, Injury to the respiratory tract by isocyanates used in making lacquers. *Brit. J. Ind. Med.*, 12 (1955) 50.

TOLOT, F., J. R. BRESSOU, V. DHERS and A. BEAUPÈRE, Manifestations pharyngées recidivantes d'origine allergique probable; rôle de la mousse de polyuréthane. *Arch. Maladies Prof.*, 22 (1961) 147.

TRENCHARD, H. J. and W. C. HARRIS, An out-break of respiratory symptoms caused by toluene diisocyanate. *Lancet*, *i* (1963) 404.

WALPOLE, A. L. and M. H. C. WILLIAMS, Toxicity of some cross-linking agents. *J. Oil & Colour Chemists' Assoc.*, 42 (1959) 694.

WALWORTH, H. T. and W. E. VIRCHOW, Industrial hygiene experiences with toluene diisocyanate. *Am. Ind. Hyg. Assoc. J.*, 20 (1959) 204.

WILLIAMS, M. H. C., Toxicity of epoxides and diisocyanates. *Chem. Age*, 41 (1959) 863.

WOODBURY, J. W., Asthmatic syndrome following exposure to toluene diisocyanate. *Ind. Med. Surg.*, 25 (1956) 540.

ZAPP, J. A., Hazards of isocyanates in polyurethane foam plastic production. *Arch. Ind. Health*, 15 (1957) 324.

9

Ethoxylin resins

PHYSICO-CHEMICAL PROPERTIES, APPLICATION

The uncured resins

An ethoxylin (= epoxy) resin together with its curing agent constitutes a two-component system. The curing ('hardening') generally ensues by *polyaddition;* by-products are not produced.

The resin component generally is called epoxy (= ethoxylin) resin after the characteristic reactive epoxy group:

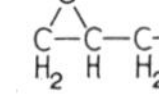

At 100° and in the presence of caustic soda a (mono- or di-) glycidyl ether is formed when epichlorohydrin is added to a polyhydroxy compound.

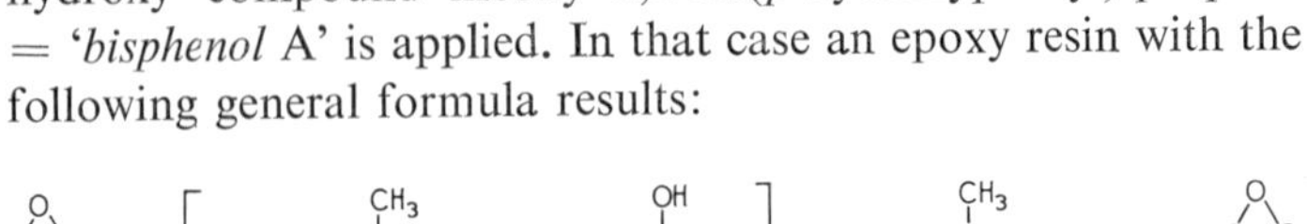

Continuing *polycondensation* produces an epoxy resin. As polyhydroxy compound mostly 2,2-bis(*p*-hydroxyphenyl)-propane = '*bisphenol* A' is applied. In that case an epoxy resin with the following general formula results:

In recent years other polyhydroxy compounds have been experimented with: glycerol, resorcinol from which glycerol–diglycidyl ethers and resorcinol–diglycidyl ethers are produced.

Each resin macromolecule possesses two epoxy groups, each of them with two active functions

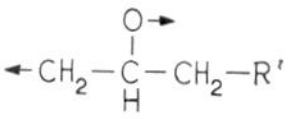

and *n* OH–R″ groups, totalling therefore 4 + *n* active functions. The *n* may vary from zero (bisphenol–diglycidyl ether) to much higher values. With increasing *n* the viscosity, the molecular weight and the number of active OH groups also increase, whereas the number of epoxy groups remains the same. The Shell-epikote resins No. 828, 1001, 1007 and 1009 for instance possess the following molecular weights: 350 to 420, 900 to 1000, 3000, 5000; the theoretical number of OH groups is 0–1, 2–3, 10, 15 (Figaret 1957).

The epoxy group must be regarded as chemically and biologically very reactive; a binding with tyrosin or lysin may be expected. With increasing viscosity, the miscibility and solubility in biological fluids decreases; in the same way the percutaneous penetration diminishes. The biological hazard, therefore, may be expected to increase with decreasing *n* and viscosity (Bourne *et al.* 1959).

The uncured epoxy resins still contain free unpolycondensated reactants; Boikina *et al.* (1960) and Shumskaja (1961) established a content of 1–10% toxic products, when heating the resins up to 60–100°: epichlorohydrin, toluene, intermediate compounds (bisepoxides, glycerol–diglycidyl ether). Shell (1958) also mentioned the presence of epichlorohydrin in all non-cured epoxy resins. In addition one has to be aware of the presence of plastifiers (*e.g.* dibutyl phthalate) or thinners (*e.g.* cellosolve, phenylglycidyl ether) in some of the delivered resins.

References p. 137

The curing agents

By reaction of the resin component with a second component, the curing agent, large macromolecular thermosetting three-dimensional structures result. The resin may react at different places (Figaret 1957):

A. in the epoxy group by:

a. polyaddition with di- or polyamines

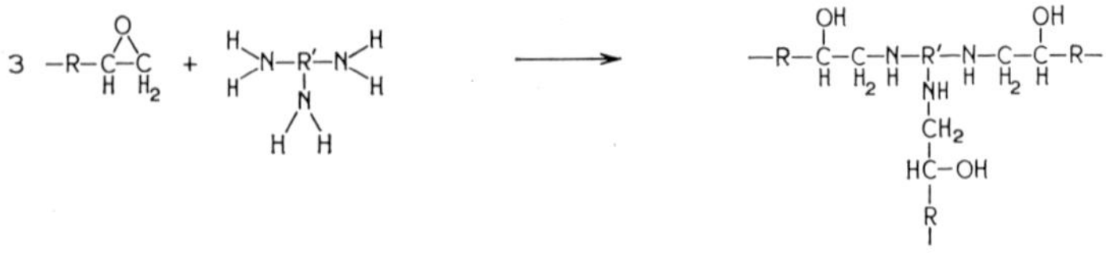

b. polyaddition with compounds carrying active OH groups (acids, alcohols, phenols)

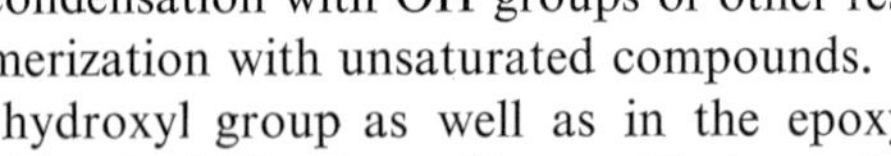

B. in the hydroxyl group by:

a. polycondensation with organic acids into polyesters,

b. polycondensation with OH groups of other resins,

c. polymerization with unsaturated compounds.

C. in the hydroxyl group as well as in the epoxy group by phthalic acid anhydride. According to Fisch *et al.* (1954) the main reaction will be as follows:

a.

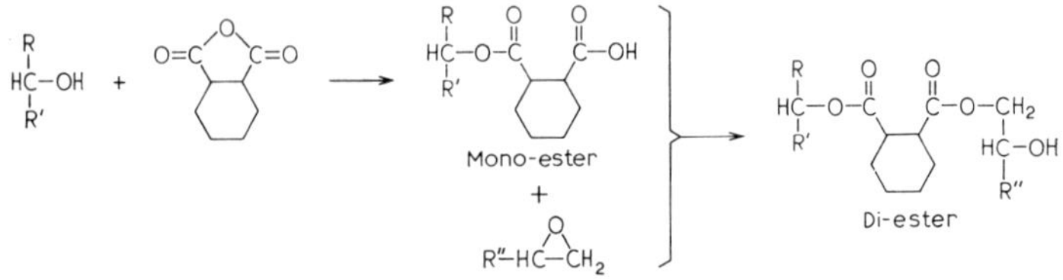

but in addition the following two etherification reactions (catalyzed by the presence of phthalic acid anhydride) are supposed to take place:

b. epoxy group directly with hydroxyl group of another resin molecule:

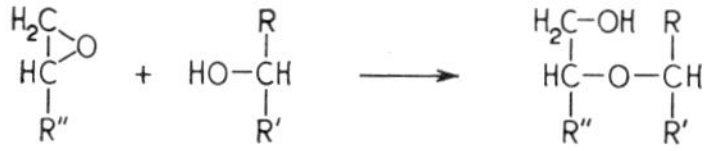

c. epoxy group directly with another epoxy group of a different resin molecule:

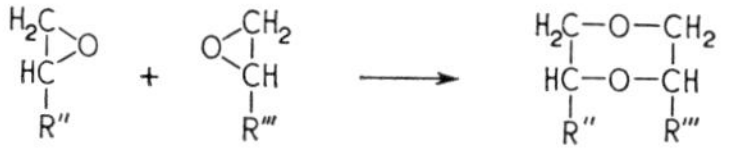

The curing agents applied in industry may be divided into:

1. acid anhydrides of phthalic acid and maleic acid. These agents are hot-curing;

2. amines, which are cold-curing and which may be divided into (Bruin 1957):

– tertiary amines, NR_3 ($R = CH_3$, C_2H_5): dimethylaminopropylamine, tris-(dimethylaminomethyl)-phenol (Narracott 1953).

– secondary amines, NHR_2: piperidine, aliphatic amines ($R = CH_3$, C_2H_5).

– polyamines, $R(NH_2)_n$, aliphatic or aromatic: ethylenediamine, diethylenetriamine (DTA), triethylenetetramine (TTA), methylenediamine, *m*-phenylenediamine. These compounds may also be applied as curing agents for resins with higher molecular weights. Particularly DTA and TTA are extensively being applied in industry.

3. polyamines from fatty acids with a surplus of ethylenediamine.

4. resins with free OH groups: pheno- and amino-plasts (Narracott 1953).

References p. 137

As several amines constitute a considerable health hazard, the industry tried to modify them in order to lower the volatility. Several modifications have been applied among which the following are mentioned:

– formation of adducts: amines modified with epoxy resins or acrylonitrile (introduction of cyanoethyl groups);

– introduction of hydroxy-alkyl groups in the NH_2: N,N′-bis (hydroxyethyl)DTA, N-(hydroxyethyl)DTA (Ingeberman *et al.* 1956; Pitt *et al.* 1957; Godard *et al.* 1958);

– modification with alkene-oxides, forming long-chain secondary amines;

– condensation products of polyamines and unsaturated fatty acids (particularly linoleic acid): Versamids (Weitgasser 1962).

In the ways mentioned above, so-called minimum-irritation-potential hardeners = MIP-hardeners are formed.

A large variety of amines may be used as hardeners. The most important representatives are the aliphatic polyamines (particularly DTA and TTA). These agents are strong alkalies; they are volatile and chemically active compounds. One may expect a biological reaction with OH groups present in amino acids; perhaps complete antigens are produced by reacting similarly with proteins (Bourne *et al.* 1959).

Methods for determination of amino acids have been proposed by English *et al.* (1944). In factories continuously processing epoxy–TTA mixtures, Grandjean (1955, 1957) never found any concentration above the lower limit of determination (150 mg/m^3) when applying this method for polyamines. In the departments investigated the evaporating surfaces, however, were relatively small (1500–3000 cm^2). This may be surpassed considerably if large objects are constructed (Zielhuis 1961).

Cured resins

Not only the two components, but also the cured resins possess some physicochemical properties of hygienic importance. Cured polyamine–epoxy resin systems may contain microscopical gas bubbles, increasing in number with increasing concentration of amine hardener. Heat curing prevents, but the presence of a plastifier promotes bubble formation. The air-free surface of blocks of cured resin are humid and rough; the pH is 12. Repeated heating makes the surface dry. The surfaces not exposed to air are dry and smooth. The cured resin (polyaddition of 10 parts epoxy resin and 1 part TTA) presumably still contains about 1% non-linked curing agent (Bourne *et al.* 1959). Bruin (1957) also established the presence of 0.5 to 8% extractable low-molecular substances in cured epikote 828 and 1001. Ideal cross-linking apparently never occurs; free NH_2 and NH groups always remain present. One of the consequences is that more than the theoretical amount of cross-linking amines has to be added.

Decomposition

The decomposition of cured epoxy resins was studied by Joyner *et al.* (1961), who observed a health hazard in the demolition of epoxy-resin concrete structures. These resins consisted of an epoxy component dissolved in xylene, the hardener component consisting of TTA and dimethylaminopropylamine. After demolition the authors established the presence of xylene, intermediate products carrying —C_6H_4—OR groups and volatile N compounds (perhaps amine hydrochloride); epichlorohydrin, free amines and chlorinated aromatic hydrocarbons could not be found.

Application

Epoxy-resin systems find application in a large variety of processes and uses: lacquer vehicles, casting resin (particularly for electric isolation), glue (particularly for joining metal and/or ceramic surfaces), glass-fibre binding compound (reinforced plastics), textile-treating agent to improve wearability and crease-resistance. The cured resins have favourable mechanical, chemical and electrical properties; they are resistant to ageing and corrosion. Casting resins may be processed like wood. Phenolformaldehyde resins can be modified with epoxy resins to yield polyalcohols used as solvents, anti-corrosives, etc. (Havris *et al.* 1954).

EXPERIMENTAL TOXICOLOGY

The non-cured resin and its components

The toxicity of epichlorohydrin proved to be considerable, because of the presence of epoxy and Cl groups. Exposure to 200 p.p.m. for a period of 4 h was lethal for rats (Carpenter *et al.* 1949). Gage (1959) determined the concentration which could be tolerated by rats during long-lasting exposure. Moderate dyspnoea, increased nasal secretion, decreased body weight, but no pulmonary edema was observed in rats and rabbits after 18 exposures to 56 p.p.m., 4 h per day. Irritation of the upper air passages was still present at 27 p.p.m., but not at 9 p.p.m. Based upon these data, Gage proposed a MAC value of 5 p.p.m. Application to the skin caused blisters; the liquid was also highly irritating to the eyes. Inhalation of 40 p.p.m. caused immediate irritation of eyes, nose and throat, but no permanent ill effects in human beings. Half of a group of unconditioned personnel detected the odor of 10–12 p.p.m. and all detected 25 p.p.m. within 5 min (Shell 1959). The proposed MAC value is below the warning level.

Very few experiments have been made on the toxicity of bisphenol A. Bornmann (1959) determined the LD_{50}-subcutaneous for rats: 2400 mg/kg (20% in propylene glycol), and the LD_{50}-oral: 4240 mg/kg. Subcutaneous implantation of 2400 mg/kg caused estrogenic effects. After sub-chronic feeding (1% in diet, 8 weeks) only decreased-growth, but no other effects were seen. The industrial hazard may be regarded as minimal (Hazlewood 1961).

In connection with the estrogenic effects of bisphenol A in rats, the following observation of Fregert *et al.* (1960) is of interest: a patient became contact-sensitized to a hair lotion. Diethylstilbestrol proved to be the offending agent. It showed a group sensitization for a great many related substances among which bisphenol A.

Many experiments have been made on the hygienic properties of uncured epoxy compounds. Epoxy resins are mixtures of relatively small molecules, each carrying two active epoxy groups; they are therefore bis-epoxides. Hendry *et al.* (1951) discovered radiomimetic and/or carcinogenic properties of some bis-epoxides, which property was not present in the mono-epoxides. Several bis-epoxides interfered with cell growth and impeded, for instance, the growth of implanted tumors. The data of Hendry *et al.* greatly stimulated the research of radio-mimetic effects of epoxy compounds, because a considerable industrial hazard might be present.

Hine *et al.* (1956) investigated the toxicity of glycidol and of some mono-glycidyl ethers in which the R was

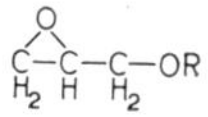

present as allyl (AGE), *n*-butyl (BGE), glycidyl (DGE), isopropyl (IGE), phenyl (PGE). These ethers are being applied as modifiers (thinners) in epoxy resins in order to decrease the viscosity. The primary toxic effect on the animal skin decreased in the following order: DGE, glycidol, PGE, AGE, BGE, IGE. Inhalation during several days caused mainly irritation of the air passages. The allyl (AGE) and the isopropyl (IGE) group produced a slight systemic intoxication. The skin effect proved to be the most important hazard, especially for DGE, glycidol and PGE. Splashed in the eyes, they may be irritating. Because of the irritant properties to the mucosa and the low volatility (b.p. above 130°) the hazard of systemic intoxication in industrial exposure may be supposed to be minimal. Moreover, the risk of skin resorption generally seems to be very small. In 1957

References p. 137

and 1958, Hine *et al.* published experimental data about the toxicity of two groups of uncured epoxy resins: an aliphatic diglycidyl ether (Epon 562) and a group of resins containing aromatic nuclei, *e.g.*, Epon 815, 820, 828, 1001, 1007 (all composed of epichlorohydrin and bisphenol) and resorcinol–diglycidyl ether (DGR). These authors determined the acute oral and intraperitoneal toxicity for rats, mice and rabbits, the local skin effect (rabbit), chronic inhalatory toxicity (rat), chronic oral toxicity (rat), local effect on rabbits' eye. The toxicity of the compounds mentioned above proved to be extremely low. Only Epon 562 and DGR (mol. wt. 300 and 222) had a slight oral toxicity, whereas the other compounds with higher molecular weights could be regarded as practically non-toxic. The LD_{50}-oral of Epon 1001 (mol. wt. 900–1000) and of Epon 1007 (mol. wt. 3000) was even more than 30 g/kg. Epon 562 and DGR were severely irritating to rabbits' eyes and skin, whereas Epon 828, 815 and 820 were moderately irritating and Epon 1001 and 1007 were non-irritating. Similar data were found by Cornish *et al.* (1959). They examined the toxicity of an uncured epoxy resin (from bisphenol and epichlorohydrin) and also two low-molecular modifiers, 2,3-epoxy-propyl ether of butanol-1 and 1,4-bis-(2,3-epoxy-propoxy)-butane. The resin had a low order of toxicity, the modifiers possessed a moderately higher toxicity, if calculated in g/kg (lower molecular weight).

Hine *et al.* (1958a, 1961a, 1961b), Walpole *et al.* (1959), Williams (1959), Kodama *et al.* (1961) paid great attention to the oncogenic and radiomimetic properties of compounds containing epoxy groups. Hine *et al.* (1958a) painted epoxy resin A (aliphatic, mol. wt. 300) and different epoxy resins B (based upon bisphenol, mol. wt. 350 to 2900) on the skin of mice over a period of 2 years (3 times a week, a 5% solution). A relatively slight oncogenic effect of epoxy resin A was observed. Intraperitoneal injection or chronic oral intake of resin A, resins B, resorcinol–diglycidyl ether (DGR, mol. wt. 224), polyallylglycidyl ether (mol. wt. 1000) or epoxidized soy-bean oil (mol. wt.

900) did not affect the frequency of pulmonary adenomata in the studied groups of mice. The authors concluded that the potential hazard of skin irritation and carcinogenesis could apparently be obviated by good industrial hygiene practice: avoidance of skin contact. Because of the extremely low volatility, no inhalatory hazard was supposed to exist. Walpole *et al.* (1959) and Williams (1959) did not observe any radiomimetic effects of epoxy resins based upon bisphenol and epichlorohydrin (the most widely used group); mono-epoxides (used as modifiers) did not affect tumor growth. Radiomimetic and/or carcinogenic effects were seen after application of glycerol-, resorcinol- and pentaerythritol-diglycidyl ether, of pentaerythritoltetraglycidyl ether and of diglycidyl adipate, whereas diglycidyl sebacate did not possess this property. Animal experiments also proved the non-carcinogenity of epoxides of oleic and linoleic acid and of squalene hexaepoxide (Van Duuren 1961), and of α_1-diepoxybutane, 9:10-epoxystearic acid, 6:7,9:10-diepoxystearic acid, whereas 1:2,3:4-diepoxybutane and 1-ethylene-oxy-3:4-epoxycyclohexane should be regarded as carcinogenic in animal experiments (Orris *et al.* 1962).

Kodama *et al.* (1961) investigated the radiomimetic properties of 13 epoxy compounds in the rat: daily intramuscular injections for a period of 3 days, repeated after a rest period of 4 days; the animals were killed on the 12th day. The authors examined the leucocyte count, the histological pattern of the liver and the number of cells in the bone marrow. In the group of mono-epoxides, glycidol (100 mg/kg), *n*-butylglycidyl ether (400 mg/kg), phenylglycidyl ether (400 mg/kg) did not cause any deviation, whereas allylglycidyl ether (400 mg/kg) and glycidyl aldehyde (50 mg/kg) caused leucopenia. In the group of bis-epoxides butadienedioxide (25 mg/kg) and diglycidyl ether (25 mg/kg) caused leucopenia, and vinylcyclohexene-dioxide (400 mg/kg) induced leucopenia and deviations in liver and bone marrow. The other bis-epoxides glycidyl-phenyl-glycidyl ether (200 mg/kg) and epoxy resin B (mol. wt. 350; 800 mg/kg) did not cause

References p. 137

any effect. In the group of tri-epoxides, diglycidyl-phenylglycidyl ether (200 mg/kg) and epoxy resin A (glycidyl-O-R-O-glycidyl; R consists of aliphatic radicals with mol. wt. 100; 100 mg/kg) did not cause any abnormality, whereas triglycidyl phosphate (25 mg/kg) and epoxy resin A in high dosage (200 mg/kg) produced leucopenia and a decreased number of bone marrow cells. From these data it may be concluded that mono-epoxides have a much lower radiomimetic effect compared to bis- and tri-epoxides. The industrial hazard of compounds with radiomimetic effects in doses up to 100 mg/kg seems to be negligible. The most widely used epoxy resin (B) once again proved to be to all intents and purposes non-toxic.

Hine *et al.* (1961a) examined the hygienic properties of diglycidyl ether (DGE) once more (see Hine *et al.* 1956). The compound proved to be corrosive for skin and subcutaneous tissue; corneal opacity occurred after skin application or inhalation (rabbit, 24 p.p.m.). Repeated exposure of rats to 3 p.p.m. caused leucopenia and depression of the bone marrow; the radiomimetic effect was apparently much stronger than that of epoxy resin A. The authors strongly advised protection of the workers from contact with DGE (liquid or vapour) and periodical examination of the exposed workers. Epoxy resin A was shown to be resorbed through the skin: 1 time 8 g/kg or 20 times 4 g/kg caused a slight leucopenia in the rat. Intramuscular and intravenous injections in rabbits and dogs had similar effects. Some of the compounds were studied more extensively regarding the hazard to the eyes. Diglycidyl ether (DGE) and diepoxybutane caused a keratitis and/or iritis in rabbits' eyes, if these animals were exposed to 24 p.p.m. and 12 p.p.m. respectively for a period of 4 h (Mettier *et al.* 1962).

The toxicity of glycid aldehyde was also studied more fully (Hine *et al.* 1961b) than previously reported (Kodama *et al.* 1961). In rats and rabbits the compound proved to be less radiomimetic than diglycidyl ether, butadiene dioxide and pentane dioxide. The strong irritative property provided a useful warning signal: exposure to even 5 p.p.m. caused unacceptable irritation of the upper air passages. A MAC of 2 p.p.m. has been proposed by the authors; however even then a periodical examination of exposed workers seemed to be desirable.

Another aspect of the toxicity of uncured epoxy resin was studied by Shumskaja (1961). She particularly emphasized the presence of volatile compounds in uncured resins. The acute oral and subcutaneous toxicity for mice of ED-5 (mol. wt. 400–450; 2–5% volatile compounds) was stronger than the toxicity of E-40 (mol. wt. 600; 4.8% volatile compounds). Chronic toxicity, however, gave different results. Exposure of rats for many months (6 days a week, 4 h per day) to vapours emanating from the resins at 80–90° caused decreased diuresis, increased electrical irritability of peripheral nerves, anemia, reticulocytosis, decreased endurance in swimming tests; in this respect the toxicity of E-40 surpassed the toxicity of ED-5. ED-5 produced 22 mg epichlorohydrin/m^3 and 6 mg toluene/m^3, whereas in the case of E-40 the concentrations were 18 and 39 mg/m^3. Shumskaja recommended a tentative MAC of 1 mg/m^3 for epichlorohydrin. Repeated application of undiluted ED-5 on rabbits' skin had a sensitizing effect. If guinea pigs were locally tested, dermatological reactions occurred earlier and more intensely, if the animals had previously inhaled the vapours for a period of one month. Resorption through undamaged skin could not be established. Ocular application of undiluted ED-5 or E-40 caused a reversible hyperemia.

Curing agents

The biological activity of the acid-curing agents phthalic and maleic acid anhydride is discussed in Chapter 6. Boron trifluoride –amine complex (hot-curing) may give rise to toxic vapours at elevated temperatures (Bourne *et al.* 1959). Boron trifluoride is very irritating to the respiratory tract; Torkelson *et al.* (1961) recommended a MAC of 0.3 p.p.m.

References p. 137

Amines

The amines are undoubtedly the most widely applied curing agents. Many amine compounds have been recommended, the toxicity of only some of them has been studied. The local effects of the amine group generally outweighs the systemic effects (Shell 1958; Eich 1960; Hofmann 1961). The primary-toxic local effect is determined by pH, concentration and type of compound: primary and secondary amines are more irritating than tertiary amines, the aliphatic compounds more than the aromatic. The last mentioned group possesses, however, the highest systemic toxicity.

The widely applied polyamine diethylenetriamine (DTA) has been investigated more fully. The LD_{50}-oral for rats is 2.33 g/kg, the LD_{50}-percutaneous for rabbits 1.09 ml/kg, whereas the primary-toxic effect on skin and eye is relatively strong. Exposure to saturated vapour for a period of 8 h did not induce death (Smyth *et al.* 1949). Application of 15% DTA (in water) caused serious corneal damage, whereas 5% solution only resulted in slight damage (Savitt 1955).

Hine *et al.* (1957, 1958b) compared the oral toxicity of 4 amines: 1,3-diaminocyclohexane proved to be moderately toxic, whereas DTA, *n*-(hydroxyethyl)-DTA (Godard *et al.* 1958) and *n*-(cyanoethyl)-DTA only possessed slight oral toxicity. At high doses, convulsions occurred. DTA possessed the strongest local effects on skin and mucosa. Cornish *et al.* (1959) also investigated the toxicity of several curing agents containing amine groups (code names). Volatility determined the inhalatory hazard to a great extent. Chronic exposure to a frequently applied compound (CD 16009 = DTA?, 19.8 mg/m^3, 7 h/day, 5 days/week, 18 weeks) did not yield any pathological effects. Except in the case of CD 16003, the acute toxicity of the curing agents was low and comparable to the toxicity of uncured epoxy resins and epoxy modifiers. A moderate-to-serious irritation of the eyes was present.

Smyth *et al.* (1944, 1949, 1951) provided range-finding toxicity data for several amines. The LD_{50}-oral for rats varied from 0.45 g/kg (2-ethylhexylamine) to 4.34 g/kg (triethylenetetramine), the LD_{50}-percutaneous for rabbits varied from 0.43 ml/kg (butane diamine) to 1.64 ml/kg (mono-isopropylamine). The primary-toxic local effects on skin and eye generally were relatively intense. Godard *et al.* (1958) also examined *n*-(hydroxyethyl)-DTA, one of the MIP-hardeners. The LD_{50}-oral for rats was 2.5 ml/kg, comparable to the LD_{50} of lactic acid; the LD_{50}-percutaneous for rabbits was 2–5 ml/kg. Inhalation of mist or vapour (produced by heating over 100°) during 2 h did not increase mortality in rabbits. Local application to the skin did not cause any effect. Application into the eyes only resulted in slight irritation. Sensibilization could not be demonstrated in guinea pigs.

Polyamides

The polyamide-hardeners (Versamid 125) are said to be relatively non-toxic; the LD_{50}-oral for rats was more than 8 g/kg. The local effects were slight, sensibilization could not be produced in guinea pigs (General Mills 1957).

Aromatic amines

Pyridine and piperidine (hexahydropyridine) possess greater systemic toxicity: liver and kidney damage (Browning 1953).

Williams (1959) and Walpole *et al.* (1959) stressed another aspect with great emphasis: some aromatic amines are well-known carcinogenic compounds. Benzidine has even been recommended as a useful curing agent. *m*-Phenylenediamine and diaminodiphenyl sulphone however are said not to be carcinogenic.

Cured epoxy resin systems

As mentioned above, the 'completely' cured resins still contain chemically active groups. Some animal experiments have been performed in order to evaluate the biological hazard of

References p. 137

these compounds. Even high doses of cured epoxy resin (50 to 75% in dioctyl phthalate) showed no acute oral toxicity for mice. Oral uptake of 1% in the diet for a period of 26 weeks only caused a decrease in body weight; no internal pathology was discovered (Shell 1954). Decreased enteric resorption may have been an important causative factor. Although Hine *et al.* (1957, 1958b) saw increased mortality in rats after feeding of 5% non-cured Epon 828 for a period of 26 weeks, the cured analogue did not cause this effect. In a laboratory experiment Petit *et al.* (1961) investigated the occurrence of subjective symptoms and objective signs caused by vapours emanating from hot-curing (110–120°) epoxy resin systems (as curing agents phthalic or tetrahydrophthalic acid anhydride were used). In 16 subjects, who had been exposed to these vapours for 1–4 years, hardly any evident objective signs and only in some cases moderate subjective feelings of irritation of the air passages could be demonstrated. The vapours were inhaled (in not recorded concentrations) during 2–3 min. The causative factor probably should be sought in the curing agents, well known irritants (see Chapter 6), and not in the uncured epoxy resin or in the cured polycondensates. Fine epoxy resin–silicon dust proved to be less fibrogenic in the intraperitoneal test in mice (0.7 ml, 1% suspension) than pure silicon (Rüttner *et al.* 1962).

EXPERIMENTAL DERMATOLOGY

Curing agents

Kydd (1960) applied one drop of undiluted diethylenetriamine on human skin: 9 out of 50 volunteers showed a reaction after 24 h which increased in the following 24 h. Fourteen days later the DTA was reapplied to the original test site. This time he found 8 positive reactions in the same 50 volunteers after 24 h. None of the 9 subjects who had reacted after the initial application showed positive reaction after reapplication 14 days later. From this, the author erroneously concluded that the 9 subjects with initial reaction had apparently become desensitized. The only valid conclusion may be that undiluted DTA has a toxic effect in 16 to 18% of the tested volunteers after 24- to 48-h skin contact, and that the 9 initially reacting volunteers appeared to be not sensitized by 48-h contact with undiluted DTA, when retested a fortnight later. Lea *et al.* (1958) compared irritant and sensitizing capacity of 4 amine curing agents, coded as CD 16005, CD 16009, CD 16019A and XH 173-50. These materials were suspended in liquid petrolatum (alcohol would have been more appropriate) and patch-tested in 25 human subjects. The patch was left in place for 48 h. The irritant concentration and the number of volunteers reacting upon these concentrations can be read in Table 4.

TABLE 4

NUMBER OF VOLUNTEERS SHOWING PRIMARY IRRITATION

Concentration	*Amine curing agents*			
%	*CD 16005*	*CD 16009*	*CD 16019A*	*XH 173–50*
100	11/25	10/25	5/5	4/25 } 1/10
10	1/25 } ½	1/25 } ½	16/25	*0/25* }
5	*0/25* }	*0/25* }	9/25	0/25
2.5	0/25	0/25	3/25 } ½	0/25
1.25	—	—	*0/25* }	—
Number of volunteers showing sensitization 14 days later, when tested with concentrations corresponding to the figures in italics:	3/25	3/25	3/25	0/25

A fortnight after the irritant tests had been completed, sensitization tests were performed. Each subject was tested with a concentration previously proven to be non-irritant. The results can be read in the last line of the table. The authors concluded '. . . XH 173-50 was the least irritating and sensitizing'. Leaving statistics and molecular weights alone, we do not agree with this conclusion about the sensitizing capacity, because in the case of XH 173-50, the challenge was applied in one-tenth of the toxic concentration, while in that of the other three compounds half of the toxic concentration was used. If these three compounds had been tested likewise at one-tenth of the toxic concentration, the number of reacting subjects would presumably have been considerably smaller, perhaps of the same order as those tested with XH 173-50. (Whether in practice curing agent XH 173-50 is less sensitizing than DTA and TTA, which are normally used, is difficult to establish. We have gathered experience in only one factory: the number of sensitized people (10 % of all workers) was about the same as observed in earlier days before introduction of XH 173-50.)

Laboratory studies reported by Ingeberman *et al.* (1956) suggested that skin irritation and sensitization by aliphatic polyamines could be modified through the introduction of selected functional groups on the nitrogen atoms. The most effective of these functional groups appeared to be the hydroxyethyl group and its alkyl and aryl derivatives. Without giving experimental details Godard *et al.* (1958) reported that in this way the primary skin-irritation potential has been greatly reduced. They performed repeated insult patch tests with a conventional polyamine hardener (unspecified) and with a substituted one (N-hydroxyethyldiethylenetriamine), both in 10% solutions in ethyl alcohol on 50 human subjects. In this procedure the same subjects are patch-tested every other day, receiving 15 applications on the same site of the skin. After a respite of 2 weeks the same individuals are challenged for sensitization by a final patch test. During the 15 applications the conventional hardener gave +++ or ++++ reactions in 35 people, whereas the low-toxicity hardener only gave +++ reactions in 2 people. In the challenging application 22 subjects appeared to be sensitized for the conventional hardener in contrast to 4 for the new MIP (minimum-irritation potential) hardener.

Epoxy compounds

In their experiments reported earlier Lea *et al.* (1958) showed the epoxy resins, code numbers CD 15003 and CD 15004B, to be toxic in concentrations of 10% and 2.5% respectively. Both resins appeared to have a sensitizing capacity: 5 volunteers of 25 tested with non-toxic concentrations reacted a fortnight later to both substances. Hine *et al.* (1958) performed prophetic patch tests on 205 human volunteers to determine their response to fabrics treated with cured epoxy resins. No irritation or sensitization has been observed.

Hine *et al.* (1956) investigated several glycidyl ethers used as viscosity reducers for epoxy resins, and observed contact sensitizations for isopropylglycidyl ether and phenylglycidyl ether. These observations might have given an answer to the question why epoxy resins have the capacity to sensitize, in other words which pattern in the chemical structure of the whole resin would be responsible for the sensitizing capacity. Hofmann (1961) worked on the same problem and concluded from animal experiments that some of the glycidyl ethers (especially phenoxypropenoxide and other cyclic epoxides) behave as outspoken sensitizers. Gaul (1957) tested one patient contact-hypersensitive to epoxy resin with butylglycidyl ether and found a negative reaction. By means of repeated insult patch tests, Klauder (1960) demonstrated the sensitizing power of bisphenoldiglycidyl ether (50% in hydrophilic petrolatum), in contrast to the cured resins. Malten (1956) reported on 13 workers sensitized for epoxy resin (Araldit D). In 5 of them he found a clear-cut positive patch test for allylglycidyl ether and one reacted to cresylglycidyl ether. Because the number of patients showing a contact sensitivity to glycidyl ethers (5) does not nearly equal 13, it seems improbable that these auxiliary substances should initiate contact hypersensitivity in those exposed to epoxy resins. These reactions upon glycidyl ethers are perhaps a sign of group-sensitization to the resin itself. Only three of 13 epoxy resin-positive patients were hypersensitive to epichlorohydrin, and two to diphenylolpropane (= bisphenol A). Sensitization for toluene or cellosolve was not revealed.

References p. 137

Gaul (1957) thought that bisphenol A was responsible for the hypersensitivity to the resin, but this is in contradiction with the just-cited findings of Malten (1956). As a matter of fact, bisphenol A can act as contact sensitizer (Fregert *et al.* 1960 and Gaul 1960), but 8 subjects with contact eczema following occupational exposure to uncured epoxy resin (Araldit), who reacted positively to tests with PVC-film containing uncured epoxy resin, were found not to react to the patch-tested bisphenol A as recently reported by Fregert *et al.* (1962). This is more or less in agreement with Malten's (1956) just-cited investigation: only 2 of 13 epoxy resin-positive persons reacted to bisphenol A.

Fregert *et al.* (1962) investigated 13 subjects *without occupational exposure* to uncured epoxy resins or epoxy hardeners who, however, on routine epicutaneous patch-testing with uncured epoxy resins (Ferroclere 900, Araldit 103, Epicote 828) reacted with allergic eczematous contact dermatitis. All of these 13 patients reacted positively to tests with epoxy resin used as a plasticizer–stabilizer in a PVC-film, and 6 of them also reacted positively to several substances belonging to the stilbestrol group. Seven of these 13 patients reacted positively to bisphenol A. In a different paper Fregert *et al.* (1962a) cite various possibilities of non-occupational contact with uncured epoxy resins: gasketing, packaging, floor tiles, coated fabrics, films, wash-proof wearing apparel, PVC gloves, PVC-handbag, PVC-chamber-pot, necklace of surface-treated beads. From these investigations one might perhaps conclude that the origin of a non-occupational contact hypersensitivity to epoxy resins can be twofold, *viz.:*

1. group-specific reaction to stilbestrol-group sensitivity (Fregert *et al.* 1960) or exposure to 'household articles' in which a surplus of bisphenol A may be present (remains to be investigated);

2. group-specific reaction to bisphenol A moiety in 'household' epoxy-resin molecules. In other words: the bisphenol A part of the 'household' epoxy-resin molecule incited the contact

hypersensitivity, but this part of the *occupationally* used resin generally does not have this capacity.

Plüss (1954) patch-tested with ethylene oxide (also a part in the resin molecule common to all epoxy resins), but obtained negative results. Just as in the case of sensitization to phenol-formaldehyde textile finish resins (see p. 50) and nylon (Jansson, 1959), it seems likely that in the majority of occupational exposure cases the low-molecular *epoxy resin structure as a whole* acts as the *primary sensitizer*, and not any special part of the resin molecule, the components of these resins, the diluents (glycidyl ethers) or the solvents. (This contradicts a suggestion of Shell 1958.) Nevertheless, Malten (1956) did observe two cases sensitized to Araldit D, who did not react upon application of several different brands of Araldit resin. In these cases solvents or added modifying substances, etc., might have acted as the actual sensitizers rather than the resin itself.

INDUSTRIAL TOXICOLOGY

Experience in industry has taught that the toxicological hazard from production and processing of epoxy resins is probably slight to moderate; the dermatological problems far outweigh the toxicological ones. Pletscher *et al.* (1954) examined 20 workers, who had been exposed to epoxy resins (based upon epichlorohydrin and bisphenol) and amine curing agents (mainly TTA). Two of them, who frequently sprayed the resin–TTA mixtures, suffered from a minor chronic bronchitis. One third of the examined group suffered from aspecific symptoms of fatigue, headache, vertigo, impotence, and in the same number of workers signs of a slight toxic hepatic disease were discovered. The authors suspected the polyamines to be responsible. One year afterwards, Breil *et al.* (1956) re-examined the same group of workers. No indication of liver disease was observed. It is not quite clear whether in the period between the two examinations exposure had remained about the same. In an electrotechnical factory, the authors examined 10 workers; this group also showed no liver pathology. Hine *et al.* (1957, 1958b) observed 250 workers from a research establishment over a period of 10 years, all of them exposed for some time (total 290 man-years) to epoxy resins. There was no indication of systemic toxicity; infrequently (24 workers) local signs of minor importance were observed: irritation of skin, eyes and upper air passages. In this establishment, however, preventive measures were more strictly observed than may be expected in normal industrial practice. Amongst 37 exposed workers, Hervieux *et al.* (1959) observed 4 cases with complaints of dizziness, anorexia, vomiting, stomach disorders; exposure to solvents, however, was also present. Zielhuis (1961) examined 50 workers from an airplane factory, exposed to epoxy resins, polyamines and sometimes also to polyester with styrene. For some of them the exposure was relatively high: large evaporating surfaces of $1\frac{1}{2}$ m^2. During an observation period of $1\frac{1}{2}$ years no evident systemic toxicity could be established, although slight aspecific complaints of drowsiness were noted. Even biochemical analysis revealed no signs of liver disease. The author concluded that the toxicological hazard from processing epoxy-resin systems in the electrotechnical industries is negligible, but against this, there was an important dermatological hazard.

Amines splashed in the eyes may cause acute painful conjunctivitis; some workers were unable to focus, while a halo-effect was observed (Savitt 1955). Several authors mentioned allergic reactions of the respiratory tract. Dernehl (1951) observed 3 cases of asthma after exposure to ethyleneamines; one of them became extremely sensitive. In 1963 Dernehl reported 8-years' experience from a department for production of aliphatic polyamines: 15 workers developed allergic asthma, but no disturbances in liver or blood were observed. In laboratory experiments with ethylenediamine (Boas-Franke *et al.* 1948) one of the authors suffered from acute coughing fits after a few weeks' exposure. Morris (1959) described allergic rhinitis and eczema in a female worker, processing epoxy resins over a period of 8 months. Another case of asthma was observed (Tolot *et al.* 1961) in a worker with a past history of acute bronchitis; this man was exposed to vapours emanating from hot-curing epoxy resins (may be acid anhydrides?). In spite of these observations asthma does not seem to constitute a serious problem. In several investigations (Pletscher *et al.* 1954; Hine *et al.* 1957, 1958b; Bourne *et al.* 1959; Zielhuis 1961) hardly any bronchitic or asthmatic syndromes were observed.

Walpole *et al.* (1959) who stressed the hazard of carcinogenic or radiomimetic effects of some epoxy compounds and amines, did not observe such reactions in workers of a laboratory or in the industry. One should bear in mind that the vapour pressures of the resins are extremely low, whereas moreover chiefly resins based upon epichlorohydrin and bisphenol have been processed in industry. The authors wisely warned against indiscriminate application of various types of epoxy resins without medical follow-up and without adequate preventive measures. This should particularly apply to resins which cause hazardous effects in animals. Possible sequelae may appear after many years of exposure. The epoxy resins have been introduced into industry relatively recently, and the time is perhaps too short for the manifestation of long-term effects.

Another aspect that should be mentioned is *decomposition.* Bergtholdt (1961) referred to complaints of odour and sickness in workers who welded or cut steel coated with epoxy-resin primer. Joyner *et al.* (1961) observed difficulties in demolishing a concrete–resin mixture. A crew of 8 workers demolished the concrete with pneumatic tools over a period of 5 days, while 4 workers sprayed the working site with water; extra ventilation was not provided for. In the first few days irritation of the respiratory tract and headache occurred. Examination of 6 workers revealed an asymptomatic albuminuria with a few cells. The causative agent could not be definitely established (see p. 107).

The industrial experience may be *summarized* as follows. The processing of epoxy resins seems to carry a slight toxic hazard, more in the field of discomfort than of real disease. The dermatological consequences outweigh the toxicological sequelae. If the former is being prevented by hygiene, ventilation, etc., the latter can also be avoided. If the low-molecular, potentially carcinogenic and/or radiomimetic resins are applied, additional care should be given to personal hygiene and medical control.

INDUSTRIAL DERMATOLOGY

Some authorities consider that the epoxies and amine hardeners are the greatest single source of contact dermatitis in industry today (Breysse 1961). In some plants using epoxies, a dermatitis rate of as high as 50% is found with sensitization occurring in approximately 10% of the exposed workers. Eich (1960) found an incidence of contact eczema in 16 of 36 workers exposed during some weeks up to two years (= 44%). Contact eczema in working up cold-setting epoxy resins was first reported by Plüss (1954) who already mentioned the case of a factory letter-carrier who became sensitized to a volatile hardener (Fluvex), without having touched any material. Three years earlier Dernehl (1951) suspected aliphatic amines to cause professional asthma and contact eczema. Pletscher *et al.* (1954) were the first to give more details. They observed 20 patients with skin manifestations on hands, forearms, face and in the genital region. They obtained positive patch tests with the resin in 6 cases, 3 of which moreover showed a positive patch to the TTA hardener; in two other patients positive patch tests were observed only for the hardener. Welcker (1955) pointed to two misleading peculiarities, *viz.*:

1. the occurrence of skin troubles in employees who did not handle the liquids themselves, but who worked at a distance of 4 m from the sites where the liquid substances were treated;
2. dermatosis often appeared first on the face (without initial involvement of the hands) and it often mimicked seborrhoic

dermatitis in localization as well as in clinical aspect. In recent years, these peculiarities have been observed less frequently, obviously due to better exhaust ventilation or to the use of less volatile substances. Moreover, conjunctivitis, paronychia and folliculitis may be seen. Grandjean (1957), investigating 11 European factories, found that 43% of all workmen dealing with the resins and amine hardeners suffered from dermatoses, and that 22% of these dermatoses were severe (3 workdays lost or change of job). Malten (1956) reported that 41 of 225 workers processing epoxy resins were, on clinical or anamnesic grounds, suspected of having contact eczema elicited by one of the ingredients used. Of the 41 suspected cases, 32 were patch-tested, in 6 cases with negative results. The remaining 26 all showed positive patch tests for epoxy resin (Araldit D). In 16 of these 26 resin hypersensitivities, a polysensitivity had developed for the hardener (Ciba hardener 951) as well. The 26 workers sensitized for the resin could be divided in two equal groups: one group applied the mixture of epoxy resin and hardener (DTA + TTA) to large objects with a large evaporation surface; in this group of 13 workers, 10 appeared to be sensitized also for the slightly volatile hardener. The other group of 13 workers applied the mixture on smaller objects; in this group only 6 workers appeared to be polysensitized for the hardener. The same ratio has been observed in other unpublished investigations and this concurs with the opinion of Hine *et al.* (1958), thus indicating the necessity of exhaust ventilation particularly in the working-up of large surfaces with (DTA + TTA)-hardeners.

Malten (1962) investigated 19 workers of an airplane factory, more or less suspected of occupational contact eczema, with 38 substances. They were engaged in working-up unsaturated polyesters or epoxy resins, a number of them, of whom 9 could be patch-tested, were exposed to both resin types. Patch tests in 4 of the 19 workers were not positive; these subjects suffered from conjunctivitis, glass-fibre dust dermatitis, dys-

References p. 137

TABLE 5

PATCH TESTS IN 15 WORKERS HANDLING EPOXY

Patient:	*1*	*2*	*3*	*4*	*5*	*6*
Araldit D, 70% acetone	–	++	++	+++	+++	++
Araldit 553, 40% acetone	–	+	++	∅	∅	+++
Araldit 430, 40% acetone	–	+	+	∅	++	+
Araldit 431, 40% acetone	–	∅	++	∅	∅	+
Epicote 828, 70% acetone	–	–	++	∅	∅	+
Hardener 951, 7% alcohol	+++	++	++	+++	–	++
Hardener DTA, 5% alcohol	∅	∅	∅	++	∅	∅
Hardener 430, 10% alcohol	+	–	–	++	+	++
Hardener 431, 10% alcohol	–	–	–	++	+	+-
Hardener 972, 10% ethyl acetate	–	+	++	±	+	+-
Hardener DMP 30, 2% ethyl acetate	–	–	–	–	–	-
Versamid 115, 10% alcohol	–	–	–	–	–	-
Versamid 140, 10% alcohol	–	–	–	–	–	-
Methyl nadic anhydride, 2% acetone	–	–	–	–	∅	-
Lamellon 6, 70% acetone	–	–	–	∅	∅	-
Lamellon 23, 70%	–	–	–	∅	–	-
Lamellon 31, 40% acetone	–	–	–	–	∅	+-
Lamellon 41 (+antimony), 40% acetone	–	–	–	–	++	-
Lamellon 51, 50% methyl ethyl ketone	–	–	–	–	–	-

ND UNSATURATED POLYESTER RESINS

7	*8*	*9*	*10*	*11*	*12*	*13*	*14*	*15*
+	+++	–	–	++	+++	–	++	++
∅	∅	–	–	∅	∅	–	∅	∅
∅	∅	–	+	+++	++	–	∅	∅
∅	∅	–	++	++	+++	–	∅	∅
∅	∅	–	+	∅	∅	–	∅	∅
+	–	–	–	+++	++	+++	–	++
±	–	∅	∅	∅	∅	∅	–	–
–	–	–	–	∅	±	++	–	+
±	+	–	–	∅	–	++	–	+
+	++	–	–	–	–	–	–	–
–	–	–	–	–	–	–	–	–
–	–	–	–	++	–	–	–	–
∅	–	–	–	++	–	+	–	–
–	∅	–	+++?	++?	–	–	–	∅
∅	∅	+	–	–	–	–	∅	∅
∅	∅	++	–	–	–	–	∅	∅
+	++	++	–	–	–	–	∅	–
+	±	++	–	–	–	–	–	–
∅	–	+	–	–	–	–	–	–

ferences p. 137

TABLE 5 *(continued)*

PATCH TESTS IN 15 WORKERS HANDLING EPOX

Tests	*1*	*2*	*3*	*4*	*5*	*6*
Lamellon 53, 40% methyl ethyl ketone	−	−	−	−	−	−
Lamellon 75, 40% acetone	−	−	−	−	−	−
Lamellon 237, 40% acetone	−	−	−	−	−	−
Laminac 4128, 40% acetone	−	−	−	−	−	−
Butanox, 1% acetone	−	−	−	++?	−	−
Palatal KR 1144, 10% acetone	−	−	−	−	−	−
Palatal P6, 10% acetone	−	−	−	−	−	−
Hobilon Z, 5% acetone	−	−	−	−	−	−
Lucidol C50,1% acetone	−	−	−	−	−	−
Trigonox K70, 0.5% acetone	−	−	−	±	−	−

hidrosis (with toenail mycosis) and eczema of unknown etiology respectively. In 12 of the 15 remaining workers (see Table 5) a contact hypersensitivity for epoxy resin (mainly Araldit D) was found, in 8 cases combined with positive patch tests for DTA + TTA (Ciba hardener 951). In 2 cases a solitary hypersensitivity for hardener 951 was revealed, and one case showed a positive patch test to unsaturated polyesters. Thus 4 cases were exclusively sensitized for the epoxy resin, 2 cases exclusively for hardener 951, and 8 showed a combined hypersensitivity to the two ingredients. Just as in 1956, resin sensitizations equalled or outnumbered the cases sensitized to the hardener. This is in contradiction to reports from manufacturers (*i.a.* Shell 1958). As far as tested, a group sensitization to different brands of epoxy resins was found in most of the cases of Araldit D hypersensitivity.

ND UNSATURATED POLYESTER (99 %) RESINS *(continued)*

7	*8*	*9*	*10*	*11*	*12*	*13*	*14*	*15*
∅	–	+	–	–	–	–	∅	–
∅	–	–	–	–	–	–	∅	∅
–	–	–	–	–	–	–	–	–
+	–	+	–	–	–	–	–	–
–	–	–	–	–	–	–	–	–
–	–	–	–	–	–	–	–	–
–	–	–	–	–	–	–	–	–
–	±	–	–	–	–	–	–	–
–	–	–	–	–	–	–	–	±
–	–	–	–	–	–	–	–	±

Several other types of hardeners also gave positive reactions in patients sensitive to hardener 951 (DTA + TTA), but workers were chiefly exposed to this type of curing agent.

In this factory about 50 workers were engaged in building hat racks, trailing edge assemblies etc. For 99 % of their weight these articles were made from unsaturated polyester resins, only 1 % of the weight was of epoxy resins which were used to glue reinforcement strips, stiffeners, etc., on the polyester body. At the moment of investigation about 12 of these 50 workers suffered from dermatoses, of which 9 could be patch-tested. Eight workers appeared to be sensitized for epoxy resin and for hardener 951, but only 5 showed a hypersensitivity to the polyester resins, 4 of which combined with a sensitization to epoxy ingredients (see Fig. 6 and the first patients in Table 5).

References p. 137

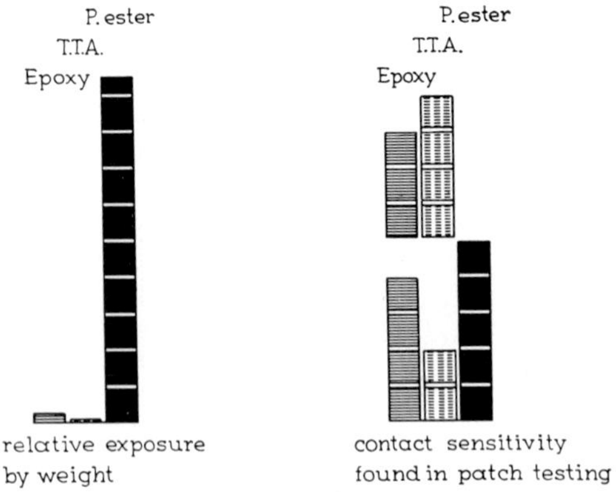

Fig. 6. Relative exposure and results of patch tests in 9 workers manufacturing hat racks with the hand-lay-up method of unsaturated polyester and epoxy resin triethylenetetramine.

Only one patient showed a sensitization to polyester exclusively. If one realizes that in the literature scarcely any reports are found on polyester sensitization and that, surveying a large polyester plant from 1955 until 1958, the author did not find a single case of polyester sensitization, then the outcome of this recent investigation in the airplane factory may perhaps be interpreted to mean that the observed sensitizations had been initiated by the epoxy ingredients and that the polyester sensitization is secondary. It should be remembered that, by weight, the exposure to epoxy ingredients only amounted to 1% of the total exposure; therefore the following advice is given. Either the whole process should be altered so as to avoid the secondary glueing of small accessory parts on the polyester body with epoxy resins, or it should be divided in two parts executed by different teams: one constructing the polyester body and the other affixing the small accessories with epoxy resins, preferably in separated workshops.

During the last year about 8 workers of the airplane factory were in intimate contact with Epikote 828 to which was added DMP 30 (2,4,6-tri-(dimethylaminomethyl)phenol) as a curing agent and methyl nadic anhydride as a modifier. This exposure mainly consisted of scraping-off surplus quantities of the semi-fluid mixture from dipped-glass roving and cleaning of the device with methyl ethyl ketone. The curing took place at about 200° in an oven, which was closed and the fumes extracted. Four men contracted occupational dermatosis during this year. We could patch-test two of them: they appeared to be sensitized to the resin only. Nevertheless the curing agent DMP 30 has been reported to be a sensitizer (Klauder *et al.* 1955). The same authors and Jirásek *et al.* (1960) reported on positive patch tests with the cured epoxy resins. Bourne (1956), Malten (1956) and Bourne *et al.* (1959) reported on sporadic cases of patients, who had become contact-sensitized, although they had handled cured epoxy resins only. This is no wonder after Bourne *et al.*'s (1959) investigation in which the unreacted amine content of an epoxy resin — TTA mixture (10:1) — even 1 year after curing, amounted to 1% of the originally added quantity of hardener. Bruno (1960) also reported on irritation of skin and mucosae on first exposure to dust of amine-cured epoxy resins; after more frequent exposure several cases of edema, papulovesicular eruption and eczema were seen.

Several cases of contact eczema in a rubber plant were traced back to the DTA and TTA content of epoxy linings of containers for latex. All these men showed polysensitization to various latex rubber ingredients, which might have been the initiators of their contact eczema, as the concentration to which they were exposed was higher than that of the leaked-out DTA + TTA (Malten 1960).

Recently, Schulz (1962) observed a crew of about 20 cable workers, of whom 4 contracted a contact eczema on their hands, fore-arms and face during the first 2–8 weeks they worked with Scotchcast Brand No. 4 Resin (M.M.M., U.S.A.) to insulate joints of cables. They all reacted positively to this resin in patch

References p. 137

tests (solutions up to 1:10,000 being positive), none reacted to the used sulphur-containing hardener.

If workers handling one type of epoxy resin become sensitized to this resin, they mostly react on patch tests with several different types and brands of epoxy resins without having had contact with the latter. Thus, among epoxy resins often a group-specificity exists (unless a reaction to identical components occurring in different brands of epoxy resins must be assumed). Malten (1956) thus reported group sensitizations in Araldit D-sensitized people with Araldit 101, 102, 103, 121 N, 553, 985 I, 985 E III, I, XV, B, F, G and Epikote 828. Recently (1962) also group-specific reactions to Araldit 430 and 431 were observed. This is a serious drawback in finding a new job assignment. This problem played probably no role with the curing agents in 1956. But recently in an airplane factory, Malten (1962) has seen among 15 plastic workers 10 cases of sensitization to hardener 951 (DTA, TTA), 6 of whom reacted to hardener 430, 6 to hardener 431, 6 to hardener 972, 1 to versamid 115 and to versamid 140. Thus a number of these patients reacted to several epoxy hardeners without having been exposed to all of them. This problem demands further investigation in cases with a clear-cut monovalent exposure because of its sociomedical implications.

Other substances mentioned in connection with epoxy resins and hardeners are the following agents patch-tested by Malten (1956) in 13 patients hypersensitive to Araldit D, 9 of whom also reacted to hardener 951:

Cyclohexanol (0/12 positive)
Cyclopentadiene (4/13 positive)
Dibutylphthalate (0/13 positive; one case reported by Jirásek *et al.* 1960).
Dioctylphthalate (1/13 positive)
Tricresylphosphate (0/7 positive)
Decaline (0/13 positive)
Toluene (0/7 positive)
Xylene (0/7 positive)
Ethyldiglycol (4/12 positive)
Methylglycol (1/13 positive)
Polyamide 115 (8/13 positive)
Thiokoll LP33 (1/13 positive)

(see for glycidyl ethers, epichlorohydrin and diphenylolpropane, p. 119).

To our knowledge sensitizations to cellosolve, *m*-phenylene diamine, piperidine, HET anhydride have not so far been reported.

We agree with Birmingham (1959) who, in an excellent review, states that only epoxy resins of lower molecular weight have irritant properties (rather liquid batches of epoxy resin may be mixed with viscosity reducers of which we know that at least allylglycidyl ether and cresylglycidyl ether are remarkably irritant to the human skin). Almost all of the amine hardeners are irritants. Their high pH (13–14) damages the keratin, and surface lipid is readily removed. Further insult follows from contact with ketone solvents used for washing and cleaning the hands, and finally alkaline industrial cleansers break the barrier, causing marked redness and dryness of the skin and thus paving the way to sensitization to hardener or/and resin. The spicules of the widely used fibre-glass play an additional role in this respect.

In a recent article, Key *et al.* (1961) mentioned a number of more recently developed ingredients of epoxy resin systems with regard to their effect on skin. They state: 'Epoxy resins may be modified with other resins for improved characteristics. Modifiers include polyamides, amino resins, phenolic resins, furanes and polysulfide liquid polymers . . . Polyamides and polysulfide liquid polymer were weak primary irritants on rabbits, but there are no reports of contact dermatitis from these agents. . . . uncured furanes can produce either irritant or allergic contact dermatitis. Less irritating curing agents have been developed for epoxy resins. These include . . . acrylonitrile–amino adducts . . . Other components of epoxy resins are . . . reactive diluents such as phenylglycidyl ether, allylglycidyl ether, butylglycidyl ether, styrene oxide, acetonitrile, styrene and aliphatic diepoxide, many of which are irritants and sensitizers'.

From a recently published article by Weitgasser (1962) it can be learned that the versamids contain a number of amide bonds and a number of free primary and secondary amino groups. This author observed one case of contact sensitivity to versamid.

References p. 137

Malten (1962) observed a group specificity in a patient sensitized for DTA + TTA (see Table 5, p. 126). At the moment of investigation the versamids had not yet been used. Patch-testing was done to evaluate eventual group-specificity to DTA + TTA hardener. In 10 cases of sensitization to this hardener, versamid 115 and 140 gave only one positive patch test each. Thus replacing this hardener by versamids may open a new perspective.

SPECIFIC PREVENTION

The necessity of the use of epoxy-resin systems for a certain purpose should be discussed between the engineers and the medical officers. If it seems impossible to use other resin systems (for instance unsaturated polyester resins) the question whether MIP (minimal-irritation potential) hardeners (or versamids?) can fulfill the requirements, should be discussed.

If the use of epoxy-resin systems seems inevitable, the question of *mechanizing* the whole work or part of it should be considered. In the manufacture of large series of electrical appliances (switch boxes, transistors) mechanization has greatly helped in lowering the incidence of contact eczema. If, however, the series are too small or the pieces of work too large, the epoxy work must be handled separately at the workshop, and the workers handling epoxy-resin systems should not be allowed to touch other materials. In this way, the spread of contaminants through tools, etc., is checked, and on the other hand the epoxy workers are not unduly exposed to other toxic or sensitizing agents, for instance solvents, or to glass-fibre spicules.

As the more liquid types of epoxy resins, the aliphatic polyamine hardeners and some of the other hardener types are primary irritants as well as contact sensitizers, *skin contact* should be avoided by all possible means. The fumes of a number of hardeners are irritating and should therefore be *locally exhausted.* Good practice requires a face velocity of not less than 30 m/min (*Hygienic Guide* 1958). This applies in particular to the fumes of aliphatic polyamines, which, moreover, may give rise to primary contact sensitization. During the mixing of resins with hardeners and additives, the temperature of the mixture may rise considerably, increasing the hazard of fume development. We therefore advise the installation of a well-ventilated '*mixing kitchen*', in which the different types of chemicals can be stored on work-bench level in closed tanks, with taps at their bottoms. Quantities just large enough for a certain task should be mechanically mixed on request in the 'kitchen' in disposable paper cups under local exhaust (also to carry-away dust from fillers) and distributed from there. In applying the resin mixture on the glass cloth, spatules or brushes with long handles should be used to obviate direct contract. The work-benches should be covered with disposable paper sheets, and the working areas should be demarcated with adhesive paper tapes. The workers should wear impermeable sleeves and aprons which may be rubbed in with a separating agent before starting work. Whenever possible, gloves of rubber or neoprene should be worn during the short periods when skin contact is inevitable. Minor contamination inside the gloves may be very dangerous, because accumulation of perspiration in the gloves enhances the wetness and thus the penetrability of the skin. It is imperative that clothing contaminated with aliphatic polyamines be removed promptly and laundered before re-use. Clothes can be removed under the shower. Flushing the skin with large amounts of running water, and washing it with mild detergent and water should be continued for at least 15 minutes.

If the skin is contaminated with resin–hardener mixture, this must be removed locally with a piece of cotton wool moistened with equal parts of acetone and alcohol or methyl ethyl ketone. This procedure may be repeated once or twice. Washing the skin in solvents should be avoided. After local removal of the contamination, the skin may be washed with an acid-type hand cleanser and dried in disposable paper towels. This should always be done before using the water closets and before work

References p. 137

breaks. After drying the skin, it may be rubbed with an acid, non-mineral grease-containing ointment. A barrier cream which should be effective against the resins as well as against the hardeners is unknown to us. Such a very thin ointment layer cannot protect regions of the skin exposed to mechanical factors connected with the work. Petrolatum may be rubbed under the nails after washing the hands, to prevent solvent and resin accumulation. If the hardeners are volatile the face should be protected with a barrier cream (for instance Kerodex BD6) particularly in the region of the eyelids. Machining cured-out epoxy resins has to be done in well-ventilated rooms, the dust locally exhausted, particularly if the resin contains glass fibres. Some of this work can be done after wetting with water in order to prevent the generation of heat and dust.

Equipment should not be used for other operations unless thoroughly cleaned with solvents (methyl ethyl ketone). For this work, heavy-duty rubber gloves must be worn.

Malten (1956), Grandjean (1955, 1957), Breysse (1960) and Eich (1961) systematically described the relevant preventive measures. Kingsley (1958) reported a reduction of skin troubles in 2/3 of the workers to about zero by observing the measures discussed above.

Measures for prevention and first aid are also described in *Chemical Safety Data Sheet* SD-76 (1959) for DTA, and in the *Hygienic Guides* (1960, 1961, 1958) for DTA, epichlorohydrin and epoxy resins. The *ACGIH* (1962) suggested the following MAC values for some of the components:

allylglycidyl ether	10 p.p.m.	=	45 mg/m^3
n-butylglycidyl ether	50 p.p.m.	=	270 mg/m^3
diglycidyl ether	10 p.p.m.	=	55 mg/m^3
glycidol	50 p.p.m.	=	150 mg/m^3
isopropylglycidyl ether	50 p.p.m.	=	240 mg/m^3

REFERENCES

American Conference Governmental Industrial Hygienists, *Threshold Limit Values*, Detroit, Michigan, 1962.

BERGTHOLDT, C. P. I., Recent welding practice at naval facilities. *Arch. Environ. Health*, 2 (1961) 257.

BIRMINGHAM, D. J., Clinical observations on the cutaneous effects associated with curing epoxy resins. *Arch. Ind. Health*, 19 (1959) 365.

BOAS-FRANKE, S. G., E. M. DRESEL and I. G. C. DRIJDEN, Properties of ethylenediamine. *Nature*, 162/4129 (1948) 960.

BOIKINA, B. S. and E. A. PEREGUD, On the presence of free epichlorohydrin in epoxide resins and quantitative methods. *Gigiena Truda Prof. Zabolevaniya*, 4 (1960) 40. Ref.: *Bull. Hyg.*, 36 (1961) 127.

BORNMANN, G. and A. LOESER, Monomer–Polymer; Studie über Kunststoffe aus ε-Caprolactam oder Bisphenol. *Arzneimittel-Forsch.*, 9 (1959) 9.

BOURNE, L. B., Medical problems associated with epoxide resins. *Trans. Assoc. Ind. Med. Officers*, 6 (1956) 94.

BOURNE, L. B., F. J. M. MILNER and K. B. ALBERMAN, Health problems of epoxy resins and amine-curing agents. *Brit. J. Ind. Med.*, 16 (1959) 81.

BREIL, H. and P. KRÖPFLI, Untersuchungen zur Frage der Leberschädigungen durch Aethoxylin-Giessharze und deren Härter. *Z. Unfallmed. Berufskrankh.*, 49 (1956) 251.

BREYSSE, P. A., Plastics in automobile body repair shops. *Ind. Med. Surg.*, 30 (1961) 141.

BROWNING, E., *Toxicity of Industrial Organic Solvents*, H.M.S.O., London, 1953.

BRUIN, P., Chemical reactions involved in the curing of epoxide–amine systems and their significance for various applications. *Lecture Fatipec Congress, Zürich*, 1957, p. 155.

BRUNO, L., Le resine epossodiche. *Med. Lavoro*, 51 (1960) 220.

CARPENTER, C. P., H. F. SMITH and U. C. POZZANI, The assay of acute vapor toxicity and the grading and interpretation of results on 96 chemical compounds. *J. Ind. Hyg.*, 31 (1949) 343.

Chemical Safety Data Sheet SD-76, *Diethylenetriamine*, Manufact. Chemists' Assoc., Washington, 1959.

CORNISH, H. H. and W. D. BLOCK, The toxicology of uncured epoxy resins and amine-curing agents. *Arch. Ind. Health*, 20 (1959) 390.

DERNEHL, C. U., Clinical experiences with exposure to ethylene amines. *Ind. Med. Surg.*, 20 (1951) 541.

DERNEHL, C. U., Hazards to health associated with the use of epoxy resins. *J. occup. Med.*, 5 (1963) 17.

EICH, J., Arbeitssicherheit beim Umgang mit Zweikomponenten-Kunststoffen. *Zbl. Arbeitsmed.*, 10 (1960) 205.

ENGLIS, D. T., and H. A. FIESS, Conduct of amino acid in synthetic ion exchangers. *Ind. Eng. Chem.*, 36 (1944) 604.

FIGARET, J., Considérations sur la constitution et les propriétés chimiques des résins époxy. *Lecture Fatipec Congress, Zürich*, 1957, p. 171.

FISCH, W. and W. HOFMANN, Über den Härtungsmechanismus der Aethoxylinharze. *J. Polymer Sci.*, 12 (1954) 497.

FREGERT, S. and H. RORSMAN, Hypersensitivity to diethylstilbestrol. *Acta Dermato-Venereol.*, 40 (1960) 206.

FREGERT, S. and H. RORSMAN, Hypersensitivity to epoxy resins with reference to the role played by bisphenol A. *J. Invest. Dermatol.*, 39 (1962) 471.

FREGERT, S. and H. RORSMAN, Hypersensitivity to epoxy resins used as plasticizers and stabilizers in polyvinylchloride (PVC) resins. *Acta Dermato-Venereol.*, 43 (1963) 10.

GAGE, J. C., The toxicity of epichlorohydrin vapour. *Brit. J. Ind. Med.*, 16 (1959) 11.

GAUL, E., Sensitizing structure in epoxy resins. *J. Invest. Dermatol.*, 29 (1957) 311.

GAUL, E., Sensitivity to bisphenol. *Arch. Dermatol.*, 82 (1960) 1003.

General Mills. *Report on non-toxicity of versamid polyamide resins, Kankakee* Ill, 1957. Ref.: BOURNE *et al.*, 1959.

GODARD, B. E., T. W. NALE, C. F. PITT and A. K. INGEBERMAN, Epoxy hardeners with low irritation potential. *Reinforced Plastics*, 2 (1958) 11.

GRANDJEAN, E., Das Risiko von Dermatosen durch kalthärtende Aethoxylinharze (Epoxydharze). *Ins. Hyg. Arbeitsphysiol. Eidgen. Techn. Hochschule, Zürich, Untersuchungsbericht*, Juli 1955.

GRANDJEAN, E., The danger of dermatoses due to cold-setting ethoxylin resins (epoxide resins). *Brit. J. Ind. Med.*, 14 (1957) 1.

HAVRIS, T. G., H. HORNING and H. A. NEVILLE, Résins phénol-formaldéhyde modifiées aux 1,2-epoxy. *Ind. Plastiques Mod. (Paris)*, 6 (1954) 53.

HAZLEWOOD, S. J., Industrial toxicology, the unknown. *Australian Paint J.*, (1961) 22.

HENDRY, J. A., R. F. HOMER, F. L. ROSE and A. L. WALPOLE, Cytotoxic agents: bisepoxides and related compounds. *Brit. J. Pharmacol.*, 6 (1951) 235. Ref.: BOURNE *et al.*, 1959.

HERVIEUX and TESSIER, Quelques observations d'exposition et d'intolérance aux dérivés vinyliques et aux résines éthoxyliques. *Arch. Maladies Prof.*, 20 (1959) 61.

HINE, C. H. and H. H. ANDERSON, Toxicological evaluation of epoxy resins. *Proc. XIIth Intern. Congress Occupational Health*, III, p. 268. Helsinki, 1957.

HINE, C. H., R. J. GUZMAN, M. K. DUNLAP, R. LIMA and G. S. LOQUVAM, Studies on the toxicity of glycidaldehyde. *Arch. Environ. Health*, 2 (1961b) 23.

HINE, C. H., R. J. GUZMAN, J. S. WELLINGTON and H. H. ANDERSON, An investigation of the oncogenic activity of two representative epoxy resins. *Cancer Research*, 18 (1958a) 20.

HINE, C. H., J. K. KODAMA, H. H. ANDERSON, D. W. SIMONSON and J. S. WELLINGTON, The toxicology of epoxy resins. *Arch. Ind. Health*, 17 (1958b) 129.

HINE, C. H., J. K. KODAMA, R. J. GUZMAN, M. K. DUNLAP, R. LIMA and G. S. LOQUVAM, Effects of diglycidyl ether on blood of animals. *Arch. Environ. Health*, 2 (1961a) 31.

HINE, C. H., J. K. KODAMA, J. S. WELLINGTON, M. K. DUNLAP and H. H. ANDERSON, The toxicology of glycidol and some glycidyl ethers. *Arch. Ind. Health*, 14 (1956) 250.

HOFMANN, H. T., Zur Frage der Gesundheitsgefährdung durch moderne Kunststoffe und ihre Lösungsmittel. *Zbl. Arbeitsmed.*, 11 (1961) 240.

Hygienic Guide, Epoxyresin systems. *Am. Ind. Hyg. Assoc. J.*, 19 (1958) 444.

Hygienic Guide, Diethylenetriamine. *Am. Ind. Hyg. Assoc. J.*, 21 (1960) 268.

Hygienic Guide, Epichlorohydrin. *Am. Ind. Hyg. Assoc. J.*, 22 (1961) 511.

INGEBERMAN, A. K. and R. K. WALTON, Low-toxicity aliphatic amines as cross-linking agents for poly-epoxy resins. *Lecture Am. Chem. Soc.*, Division of paint, plastics and printing ink chemistry, 1956.

JANSSON, H., Zur Frage der Sensibilisierungseigenschaft von Perlon und Nylon-Grundsubstanz. *Z. Haut. Geschlechtskrankh.*, 26 (1959) 37.

JIRASEK, L. and J. KALENSKY, Epoxy resins. *Pracovni. Lekar.*, 12 (1960) 67. Ref.: *Berufsdermatosen*, 8 (1960) 286.

JOYNER, R. E. and W. L. PEGUES, A health hazard associated with epoxy resin concrete dust. *J. Occupational Med.*, 3 (1961) 211.

KEY, M. M., V. B. PERONE and D. J. BIRMINGHAM, Patch-testing in dermatitis from the newer resins. *J. Occupational Med.*, 3 (1961) 361.

KINGSLEY, W. H., Health hazards and control of an epoxy resin operation. *Am. Ind. Hyg. Assoc. J.*, 19 (1958) 258.

KLAUDER, J. V., Patch-test study to determine cutaneous reaction to new compounds. *Arch. Environ. Health*, 1 (1960) 407.

KLAUDER, J. V. and F. C. COMBES, Aspects of occupational dermatoses. *Ind. Med. Surg.*, 24 (1955) 13.

KODAMA, J. K., R. J. GUZMAN, M. K. DUNLAP, G. S. LOQUVAM, R. LIMA and C. H. HINE, Some effects of epoxy compounds on the blood. *Arch. Environ. Health*, 2 (1961) 50.

KYDD, W. L., Toxicity evaluation of diethylenetriamine. *J. Dental Res.*, 39 (1960) 46.

LEA, W. A., W. P. BLOCK and H. H. CORNISH, The irritating and sensitizing capacity of epoxy resins. *Arch. Dermatol.*, 78 (1958) 304.

MALTEN, K. E., *Beroepsekzeem bij het verwerken van kunststoffen*, Thesis, Amsterdam, 1956.

MALTEN, K. E., Unpublished data, 1960.

METTIER, S. R., H. K. BOYER, W. K. MCEWEN, F. IVANHOE, F. H. MEYERS and C. H. HINE, Effects of air-pollutant mixtures on the eye. *Arch. Environ. Health*, 4 (1962) 103.

MORRIS, G. E., Allergic rhinitis acquired during the processing of epoxy resins. *Ann. Allergy*, 17 (1959) 74.

NARRACOTT, E. S., The curing of epoxide resins. *Brit. Plastics*, 26 (1953) 120.

ORRIS, L., B. L. VAN DUUREN and N. NELSON, Carcinogenity of oxy compounds, *VIIIth Intern. Cancer Conference*, Moscow, 1962.

PETIT, J. M., J. TROQUET and J. MELON, Influence des émanations provenant des manipulations de résines éthoxylines sur les voies respiratoires. *Arch. Maladies Prof.*, 22 (1961) 718.

PITT, C. F. and M. N. PAUL, Low-toxicity aliphatic amines for cross-linking poly-epoxy resins. *Mod. Plastics*, 34 (1957) 125 and 202.

PLETSCHER, A., R. SCHÜPPLI and R. REIFERT, Über Gesundheidsschäden durch Giessharze. *Z. Unfallmed. Berufskrankh.*, 47 (1954) 163.

PLÜSS, J., Ekzem durch neue Kunstharze. *Z. Unfallmed. Berufskrankh.*, 47 (1954) 83.

RÜTTNER, J. R., R. RONDEZ, H. BÜHLER and A. STOFER, Zur Frage der fibrogenetischen Wirkung eines gewerblichen Araldit-staubgemisches. *Z. Unfallmed. Berufskrankh.*, 55 (1962) 24.

SAVITT, L. E., Contact dermatitis encountered in production of epoxy resins. *Arch. Dermatol. Syphilol.*, 71 (1955) 212.

SCHULZ, K. H., personal communication (1962).

Shell Chemical Corp., Epoxy resins in industry. *Ind. Accident Prevention Bull.*, 26 (1958) 280.

Shell Chemical Corp., *Technical Bulletin*, May, 1954. Ref.: BOURNE *et al.*, 1959.

Shell Chemical Corp., Epichlorohydrin. *Ind. Hyg. Bull.*, SC 57-86. Ind. Hyg. Dept., New York, 1959. Ref.: Hygienic guide. *Am. Ind. Hyg. Assoc. J.*, 22 (1961) 511.

SHUMSKAJA, N. I., Toxicological characteristics of some epoxy resins. *Gigiena Truda i Prof. Zabolevaniya*, 5 (1961) 34.

SMYTH, H. F. and C. P. CARPENTER, The place of the range-finding test in the industrial toxicological laboratory. *J. Ind. Hyg.*, 26 (1944) 269.

SMYTH, H. F., C. P. CARPENTER and C. S. WEIL, Range-finding toxicity data. List III. *J. Ind. Hyg.*, 31 (1949) 60.

SMYTH, H. F., C. P. CARPENTER and C. S. WEIL, Range-finding toxicity data. List IV. *Arch. Ind. Hyg.*, 4 (1951) 119.

TOLOT, F., M. COLIN and R. SOUBRIER, Asthme et araldite. *Arch. Maladies Prof.*, 22 (1961) 163.

TORKELSON, T. R., S. E. SADEK and V. K. ROWE, The toxicity of boron trifluoride when inhaled by laboratory animals. *Am. Ind. Hyg. Assoc. J.*, 22 (1961) 263.

VAN DUUREN, B. L., Separation and identification of aliphatic and aromatic carcinogens from environmental sources, *Symposium on Analysis of carcinogenic air pollutants*, Cincinnati, August 1961.

WALPOLE, A. L. and M. H. C. WILLIAMS, Toxicity of some cross-linking agents. *J. Oil Colour Chemists' Assoc.*, 42 (1959) 694.

WEITGASSER, H., Untersuchungen über die hautreizende Wirkung neuer Versamid-Epoxyharz-Verbindungen. *Berufsdermatosen*, 10 (1962) 134.

WELCKER, A., Gewerbeekzem durch Arbeit mit Giessharz. *Dermatol. Wochschr.*, 33 (1955) 871. Ref.: *Zbl. Arbeitsmed.*, 5 (1955) 96.

WILLIAMS, M. H. C., Toxicity of epoxides. *Chem. Age*, 41 (1959) 863.

ZIELHUIS, R. L., Systemic toxicity from exposure to epoxy resins, hardeners and styrene. *J. Occupational Med.*, 3 (1961) 25.

ZSCHUNKE, E., Über die Epoxydharz-Dermatitis. *Deut. Gesundheitsw.*, 14 (1959) 1810. Ref.: *Zbl. Arbeitsmed.*, 10 (1960) 247.

10

Vinyl polymers

PHYSICO-CHEMICAL PROPERTIES, APPLICATION

By substitution of different groups in ethene (= ethylene, $CH_2{=}CH_2$), the tendency to polymerization increases. These substituted monomers are called *vinyl compounds* ($CH_2 = CHR$). The polymerization proceeds by opening of unsaturated bonds; no by-products and no intermediates are formed. Relatively large quantities of auxiliary substances, particularly plasticizers, may be applied. The end-products are thermoplastic linear macromolecules. The production of polymers generally proceeds in closed systems; the processing of the polymer end-products (mostly as granules or powders) into consumer goods, for instance by extrusion, takes place in the polymer phase: heat-moulding of the thermoplast into the desirable shape. The auxiliary substances are added to the polymerizates in a physical mixing process.

Huge quantities of vinyl compounds have been produced and processed in the last decades. An enormous variety of plastic consumer goods belongs to this group of thermoplasts.

The most important vinyl polymers are:

Polyvinyl chloride (PVC)

The monomer vinyl chloride ($CH_2{=}CHCl$) is produced from acetylene (C_2H_2) and Cl_2 under high pressure with Hg

References p. 152

salts as catalysts or from 1,2-dichloroethane at 400°. (An epidemic of Hg-intoxication was reported in Japan amongst fishermen; the cause was the Hg-effluent of a PVC factory (Kurland *et al.* 1960). Polymerization usually takes place in an emulsion phase; from the dried polymerizate a great variety of rigid objects made, but also foils, soft plastics and foam plastics. The products may be welded at about 200°. By conducting Cl_2 through a suspension of PVC in tetrachloroethane (a highly toxic solvent) chlorinated PVC (PeCe) may be formed. Vinylchloride is also widely applied as copolymer, for instance with PV acetate or with acrylonitrile.

Polyvinyl esters

e.g. PV acetate and PV propionate, produced from C_2H_2 and the corresponding acid with Hg, Cd, Pb or Zn salts as catalysts. They may be applied as binder in lacquers, as glue or as chewing gum.

Polyvinyl alcohol

is produced by hydrolysis of the PV esters; the monomer vinyl alcohol ($CH_2{=}CHOH$) as such does not exist. The polymer is soluble in water; bichromates may be added to decrease this solubility.

Polyvinyl acetals

are produced from PV alcohol and aldehydes, for instance formaldehyde (PV formal).

Polyvinyl ether

is produced from C_2H_2 and alcohol or from vinyl chloride and alkali alcoholate; boron trifluoride may be used as catalyst.

Polyvinylidene chloride

From vinyl chloride and Cl_2 a (toxic) chlorinated hydrocarbon 1,1,2-trichloroethane is formed, which is transformed into vinylidene chloride ($CH_2{=}CCl_2$), a monomer usually applied in copolymerization.

Polystyrene

is produced from vinylbenzene (= styrene, $CH_2=CH-C_6H_5$). The monomer styrene is polymerized as such (decaborane, $B_{10}H_{14}$, may be used as accelerator), or as copolymer especially in synthetic rubbers (Buna-S, Buna SS and so on). Regarding its use as a cross-linking agent in unsaturated polyesters, see Chapter 7, p. 72.

Polyfluoroethylene, see Chapter 12, p. 172.

Polyacryl derivatives, see Chapter 11, p. 155.

Decomposition

of PVC and other Cl-containing polymers at 300° may yield HCl, CO and CO_2; about 30% of the Cl content may be lost as HCl. In a non-ventilated room of 1000 ft³, the burning of about 3 lb plastic may constitute a real toxic hazard, although the HCl production gives a good warning signal by irritation (Coleman *et al.* 1954); phosgene does not occur. Burning of PVC-coated laminated wood increases the CO concentration (Schriesheim 1956).

EXPERIMENTAL TOXICOLOGY AND DERMATOLOGY

Mastromatteo *et al.* (1960) exposed rats, mice and guinea pigs to 10, 20, 30 or 40 vol.% vinyl chloride in air; narcosis and death occurred in mice and rats after 30-min exposure to 30% vinyl chloride, guinea pigs were somewhat less sensitive. On autopsy pulmonary congestion and edema, congestion of liver and kidney and decreased clotting of the blood were found. Based upon previous experiments reported by these authors and upon their own data, they judged a concentration of 500 p.p.m. (= 1300 mg/m³) to be acceptable for industry. But long-lasting experiments reported later by Torkelson *et al.* (1961) raised doubt as to the acceptability of this value. Rabbits, rats, guinea pigs and dogs were exposed for 4½ to 6 months, 5 days per week, 7 h per day to 500 p.p.m. (only in rats),

200 p.p.m., 100 p.p.m. or 50 p.p.m. Repeated exposure to 500 p.p.m. vinyl chloride caused increased central lobular degeneration in the liver and interstitial and tubular changes in the kidney; exposure to 100 p.p.m. still gave rise to an increased weight of the liver in rats. The highest concentration without any effect in all these animals after repeated exposure was 50 p.p.m. Torkelson *et al.* therefore proposed a maximum allowable average concentration of 50 p.p.m. with a maximum peak concentration of 100 p.p.m.

Carpenter *et al.* (1949) reported on the toxicity of vinylidene chloride and vinyl acetate; 2 to 4 of 6 rats died after exposure for 4 h to 32,000 p.p.m. and 4,000 p.p.m. respectively. Vinyl acetate is said to have no important health hazards (*Chemical Safety Data Sheet* SD-75, 1959).

Schulz (1962) sensitized about 70% of a group of 100 guinea pigs by daily epicutaneous application (during 4–7 days) of 0.1–0.5% monovinylcarbazole dissolved in equal parts of alcohol and ol. olivarum. Electricians may get 'dermatitis' from vinylcarbazole used for insulation (Schwartz *et al.* 1957).

The toxicity of pyrolysis products of PVC and of isocyanate foam plastic were compared by Zapp (1957); the results were similar for both plastics. Decomposition at 200° caused death in 2 of 4 rats after an exposure of 6 h, whereas the emanating pyrolysis products at 560° caused death in 1 of 2 rats after 10 min; the cause of death was pulmonary edema.

Regarding the toxicity of vinylbenzene = styrene, see Chapter 7, p. 73.

INDUSTRIAL TOXICOLOGY

Although polyvinyl polymers are produced and processed in huge quantities, industrial-hygienic complications appear relatively very seldom in the literature. This may be explained as follows (see Chapters 1 and 2):

– Generally the monomers are not very toxic (exceptions!);

- The polymerization to a final high-polymer end-product ensues in closed systems; by-products and intermediates are not formed;
- The processing and also the mixing with auxiliary substances ensues in the high-polymer, biologically inactive phase.

The production of PVC has given rise to a number of intoxications caused by the monomer. Dublin *et al.* (1933, 1941) reported two slight intoxications in workers exposed for about 3 min to 2–5% vinyl chloride: reversible vertigo, light disorientation and burning feeling in the feet. Two more serious cases were reported in the *Annual Report of the Chief Inspector of Factories* in Great Britain (1953): collapse after exposure of 10 min with aspecific symptoms during recovery in a worker who stood near an open polymerization tank, and in a maintenance worker during repair of a leak. Three cases of intoxication, two of them fatal, were described by Danziger (1960) from Canada. One worker died while cleansing a tank for 10 min; the cause of death could not be definitely established. Another worker became fatally drowsy when working near an open valve of a vinyl chloride tank (decreased blood clotting was found); a fellow worker, coming to his rescue, became very dizzy, but quickly recovered after inhaling fresh air. In the last two cases vinyl chloride definitely proved to be the causative agent. Harris (1953) mentioned a primary toxic effect on the skin: vinyl chloride may cause burns; the *Chemical Safety Data Sheet* SD-56 (1954) speaks of 'freezing'.

Filatova *et al.* (1958) reported on 'chronic angioneurosis' in workers from a PVC factory, who, however, were exposed not only to 20–315 p.p.m. vinyl chloride, but also to solvents (dichloroethane; methanol); particularly the sampling of specimens from the reaction tanks gave rise to high concentrations in air.

Apart from the above-mentioned hygienic effects reported in PVC factories, a few reports deal with workers handling the polymer. Devigneveille *et al.* (1953) mentioned digestive disorders, dermatitis and some aspecific disturbances of the peripheral blood in workers processing PVC; the data are inconclusive as to the real cause: polymer or auxiliary substances? The latter compounds were probably also responsible for acne on the forearm and face in workers handling PVC products, where chlorinated paraffins were used as plasticizer (Roubal *et al.* 1953). In 145 workers, handling several PV polymers (no data about type of plastic and about intensity of exposure) Hervieux *et al.* (1959) observed 17 subjects with skin disorders (2 cases of eczema, 10 with pruritus), gastric disorder (1 case), irritation of the mucosae (4 cases); exposure to other compounds also was present (glass-fibre materials, Pb and Co salts, acetone). Irritation was also mentioned by Parmeggiani *et al.* (1955) in workers filling bags with monomer-free PVC powder.

Quooss (1959) pointed to the occurrence of sometimes highly toxic solvents in PVC glues: dichloroethane, trichloroethylene and dioxan; he proposed substitution by the less toxic methylene chloride.

Regarding the production, processing and handling of polystyrene or styrene-copolymerizates, some authors also reported a few biological phenomena. Wilson (1944) observed in workers in a rubber factory exposed to a concentration of styrene below 500 p.p.m. irritation of eyes and air passages, asthenia and lassitude, although physical examination did not reveal any morbid symptoms. The skin was dry, rough and fissured. Baader (1960) described a lymphoblastic sarcoma of the colon with hemorrhagic diathesis in a worker exposed for 7 years to styrene–butadiene under bad war-time conditions of ventilation. This is the only report in the literature indicating effects similar to that of benzene. It may be seriously doubted whether the supposed occupational genesis was real; other experiences from industry and experimental data (see Chapter 7) do not confirm such a relationship. In this respect only a slight leucopenia with relative lymphocytosis has been reported by Italian authors (Barsotti *et al.* 1952; Parmeggiani *et al.* 1955). Prokowsky (1953) reported leucocytosis, sometimes anemia and thrombopenia in (female?) workers exposed to less than 150 p.p.m. styrene. Gastro-intestinal disorders with hypotonia have been described by Drogicina *et al.* (1959) in workers exposed for more than 5 years to styrene in a rubber factory. From a similar factory another Russian author, Katz (1962), reported the occurrence of a toxicochemical hepatitis, a disturbed serum protein pattern and a tendency to leucopenia (no data about exposure to other chemical agents such as acrylonitrile). Regarding the industrial hazard of styrene, see also Chapter 7, p. 76.

Outside the industrial field, Bergman *et al.* (1962) reported lung lesions after frequent inhalation of hair spray, which contained polyvinyl pyrrolidone. They described 15 cases, one of them in a hairdresser. The lesions usually regress with termination of exposure, but in some cases may result in fatal alveolar capillary block syndrome.

Some biological consequences have been reported from *decomposition products* of PVC plastics. In workers in a PVC factory exposed to heated polymers (160°), Tribuch (1949) observed a white coating on the mucosa of the upper air passages, chronic gastritis, liver disturbances, anemia and hypotension; chlorinated paraffins used as plasticizer probably were responsible for these signs, because also an acneiform skin disease was present. Storlazzi (1959) reported phenomena more definitely related to decomposition products of PVC: welding or cutting ship or tank constructions coated with a PVC lacquer produced very irritating vapours. HCl concentrations of 2–35 p.p.m. occurred; phosgene could not be found. He proposed to remove mechanically about 5 cm of the coating next to the welding suture before welding. Quooss (1959) stressed the same point. This author also observed irritation of mucosa and gastric disturbances when a polystyrene extruder became overheated; styrene and ethylbenzene probably caused these effects.

INDUSTRIAL DERMATOLOGY

Schwartz *et al.* (1940) reported on 'can poisoning', a sensitization dermatitis occurring in workers who had contact with dust of the inner coating of tin cans, which consisted of a vinylite resin (this is a general name for PVC, PVA, PV-butyral etc.). The coating mixture consisted of the resin, plasticizers, petroleum solvent, and a lead-free drier, and was heated for 20 min to 400° F. Three workers showed positive patch tests to the applied polymerized dust, which might be due to zinc or tin chloride generated during the heat polymerization of the resin when applied on the metal parts. Zeisler (1940) reported on two cases of sensitization (due to garters, suspenders and a wrist watch strap) after contact with copolymerizates of vinyl chloride and vinyl acetate. Hitschmann (1950) reported on contact eczema due to tablecloth of vinylplastic fabric and Kipping (1959) mentioned contact eczema from a vinylplastic tape used to repair torn textile material (there was a 2+ reaction to the laundered tape after 48-h skin contact).

Generally, PVC, PVA, etc. in themselves are considered inert (Harris 1953; Sonneck 1962) and the three cases reported above may concern the added stabilizers or plasticizers, which were not investigated separately. Schwartz (1945) reported that the actual irritants in the wearing apparel were found to be the plasticizers and stabilizers (dibutyl-tin maleate, dibutyl sebacate). He also reported on workers engaged in coating fabrics with PVC and PVA copolymer, whose dermatitis was found to be due to a by-product formed in the recovered acetone solvent during the recovery process, namely biacetyl. When this was removed the outbreak of 'dermatitis' ceased.

Sonneck (1962) patch-tested 4 contact-sensitized patients in the manufacture of PVC cables with PVC-F and PVC-G (weak positive reactions) and with the added lead montanate (clearly positive reactions). This stabilizer additive consisted of lead hydroxide, montan wax and emulgator E 30. The former two gave negative reactions, but the latter gave clearly positive reactions. This emulgator E 30 is made of mepasin (negative reactions) and a sodium salt of this raw material containing sodium salt of alkylsulfonic acid. If PVC is reacted with additional chloride one obtains PeCe, which is soluble in organic solvents. Dissolved in dichloroethane, tetrachloroethane, toluene, acetone, chlorobenzene, butyl acetate, etc., it is used as a lacquer or glue. Sonneck (1962) described in a worker who had handled these PeCe products for years, a short-lasting contact sensitization to PeCe powder tested in petrolatum with positive results. The solvents in these glues and the degreasing action of emulgator E 30 may have paved the way to these sensitizations for PeCe and PVC respectively. The same mechanism may be the basis of sensitizations seen by Raymond (1959) in workers constructing parquet floors, who used a vinyl acetate-containing adhesive. Also Gunther (1956) reported on dermatoses due to use of polyvinyl acetate, especially if not fully polymerized, or if used with irritating plasticizers.

SPECIFIC PREVENTION

The hitherto accepted MAC for vinyl chloride: 500 p.p.m. = 1300 mg/m^3 (A.C.G.I.H., 1962) probably is too high; one should take into consideration the experimental data reported by Torkelson *et al.* (1961), who proposed a MAC of 50 p.p.m. (= 130 mg/m^3) as daily average with peak concentration of 100 p.p.m. (= 260 mg/m^3). The hazard of exceeding these values in industry is relatively small. Prescriptions for handling vinyl chloride and vinyl acetate have been given by the *Chemical Safety Data Sheets* SD-56 (1954) and SD-75 (1959). For styrene, see Chapter 7, p. 75.

REFERENCES

American Conference Governmental Industrial Hygienists, *Threshold Limit Values*, Detroit, Michigan, 1962.

BAADER, E. W., *Klinische Grundlagen der sechsundvierzig meldepflichtigen Berufskrankheiten*, Urban & Schwarzenberg, München, 1960.

BARSOTTI, M., L. PARMEGGIANI and C. SASSI, Observations on occupational pathology in a polystyrene resin factory. *Med. Lavoro*, 43 (1952) 418. Ref.: *Arch. Ind. Hyg.*, 7 (1953) 358.

BERGMAN, M., I. J. FLANSE, P. T. CRUZ, N. KLAM, P. R. ARONSON, R. A. JOSLI and H. T. BLUMENTHAL, Thesaurosis due to inhalation of hairspray. *New Engl. J. Med.*, 226 (1962) 750.

CARPENTER, C. P., H. F. SMYTH and U. C. POZZANI, Assay of acute vapor toxicity and the grading and interpretation of results on 96 chemical compounds. *J. Ind. Hyg.*, 31 (1949) 343.

Chemical Safety Data Sheet SD-56, *Vinyl chloride*, Manufact. Chemists' Assoc., Washington, 1954.

Chemical Safety Data Sheet SD-75, *Vinyl acetate*, Manufact. Chemists' Assoc., Washington, 1959.

Chief Inspector of Factories, *Annual Report 1951*, Cmd 8772, H.M.S.O., London, 1953. Ref.: MASTROMATTEO *et al.*, 1960.

COLEMAN, E. H. and C. H. THOMAS, The products of combustion of chlorinated plastics. *J. Appl. Chem.*, 4 (1954) 379.

DANZIGER, H., Accidental poisoning by vinyl chloride. *Can. Med. Assoc. J.*, 82 (1960) 828.

DEVIGNEVEILLE and A. M. FLUCHER, *Étude toxicologique expérimentale des résines polyvinyliques*, Service méd. manufact. Saint-Marcel, Vernon, 1953. Ref.: TRUFFERT, 1959.

DROGICINA, E. A., G. N. MAZUNINA, A. A. ORLOWA, H. M. RASCHEWSKAJA and E. A. SOLOWIEWA, Klinik der chronischen Vergiftung bei der Herstellung von synthetischen Divinylsterol und Chloropren Kautschuk. *Gigiena Truda i Prof. Zabolevaniya*, 3 (1959) 10. Ref.: *Zbl. Arbeitsmed.*, 11 (1961) 199.

DUBLIN, L. J. and R. J. VANE, Occupational hazards and diagnostic science. *Bulletin* No. 582 (1933); *Bulletin* No. 41 (1941) *U.S.A. Dept. Labor*, Ref.: DANZIGER, 1960.

FILATOVA, V. S., L. J. BALAKHONOVA and E. GRONSBERG, Hygienic conditions in the production of vinyl chloride. *Gigiena Truda i Prof. Zabolevaniya*, 1 (1958) 6. Ref.: *Public Health Engin. Abstr.*, 40 (1960) No. 4, p. 16.

GUNTHER, O., Die Kunststoffe und ihre arbeitsmedizinische Bedeutung. *Zbl. Arbeitsmed.*, 6 (1956) 156.

HARRIS, D. K., Health problems in the manufacture and use of plastics. *Brit. J. Ind. Med.*, 10 (1953) 255.

HERVIEUX and TESSIER, Quelques observations d'exposition et d'intolérance aux dérivés vinyliques et aux résines éthoxyliques. *Arch. Maladies Prof.*, 20 (1959) 61.

HITSCHMANN, O., Contact dermatitis due to table cloth cover of vinylplastic fabric. *Arch. Dermatol. Syphilol.*, 61 (1950) 679.

KATZ, B. YA., Toxicochemical hepatitis due to styrene exposure. *Gigiena Truda i Prof. Zabolevaniya*, 6, 10 (1962) 21.

KIPPING, H. F., Dermatitis from thermoplastic tape. *Arch. Dermatol.*, 80 (1959) 348.

KLIMKOVA-DEUTSCHOVA, E., Neurologische Befunde in der Plastikindustrie bei Styrol-Arbeitern. *Intern. Arch. Gewerbepathol. Gewerbehyg.*, 19 (1962) 35.

KURLAND, L. T., S. N. FARO and H. SIEDLER, Minamata disease. *World Neurol.*, 1 (1960) 370. Ref.: *Ind. Med. Surg.*, 31 (1962) 181.

MASTROMATTEO, E., A. M. FISHER, H. CHRISTIE and H. DANZIGER, Acute inhalation toxicity of vinyl chloride to laboratory animals. *Am. Ind. Hyg. Assoc. J.*, 21 (1960) 394.

PARMEGGIANI, L. and C. SASSI, Risques et pathologie professionnelle dans la fabrication et le travail de quelques matières plastiques. *Med. Lavoro*, 46 (1955) 14. Ref.: *Arch. Maladies Prof.*, 16 (1955) 507.

PROKOWSKY, V. A., Berufsschäden bei Erzeugung synthetischen Kautschuks. *Gigiena i Sanit.*, 9 (1953) 17. Ref.: KLIMKOVA-DEUTSCHOVA, 1962.

QUOOSS, H., *Gesundheitsgefahren in der Kunststoffindustrie*, Barth, Leipzig, 1959.

RAYMOND, V., Les dermatoses des parqueteurs. *Travail et Sécurité*, 5 (1959) 186.

ROUBAL, J. and F. POKORNY, Occupational disease in the manufacture of polyvinylchloride products. *Pracovni Lekar.*, 5 (1953) 144. Ref.: WILSON *et al.*, 1960.

SCHRIESHEIM, A., A method for the controlled burning of combustible materials and analysis of the combustion gases. *J. Res. Natl. Bur. Std.*, 57 (1956) 245. Ref.: COLEMAN, 1954.

SCHULZ, K. H., personal communication (1962).

SCHWARTZ, L., Dermatitis from synthetic resins. *J. Invest. Dermatol.*, 6 (1945) 239.

SCHWARTZ, L. and J. P. RUSSELL, Occupational dermatitis from handling resin lined tin cans. *J. Am. Med. Assoc.*, 115 (1940) 448.

SCHWARTZ, L., L. TULIPAN and D. J. BIRMINGHAM, *Occupational diseases of the skin.* Lea and Febiger, Philadelphia, 1957.

SONNECK, H. J., Berufsbedingte Hautschäden durch Polyvinylchlorid. *Berufsdermatosen*, 10 (1962) 38.

STORLAZZI, E. D., Hygiene of welding in U.S. naval shipyards. *Arch. Ind. Health*, 19 (1959) 307.

TORKELSON, T. R., F. OYEN and V. K. ROWE, The toxicity of vinyl chloride as determined by repeated exposure to laboratory animals. *Am. Ind. Hyg. Assoc. J.*, 22 (1961) 359.

TRIBUCH, S. L., Polyvinylchloride. *Gigiena (Moskau)*, 10 (1949) 38. Ref.: QUOOSS, 1959.

TRUFFERT, L., Aspects toxicologiques de l'industrie des matières plastiques. *Arch. Maladies Prof.*, 20 (1959) 43.

WILSON, R. H., Health hazards encountered in a manufacture of synthetic rubber. *J. Am. Med. Assoc.*, 124 (1944) 701.

WILSON, R. H. and W. E. MCCORMICK, Plastics. *Arch. Ind. Health*, 21 (1960) 536.

ZAPP, J. A., Hazards of isocyanates in polyurethane-foam plastic production. *Arch. Ind. Health*, 15 (1957) 324.

ZEISLER, E. P. Dermatitis from elastiglass garters and wrist watch straps. *J. Am. Med. Assoc.*, 114 (1940) 2540.

11

Acrylic polymers

PHYSICO-CHEMICAL PROPERTIES, APPLICATION

Derivatives of acrylic acid polymerize by opening of double bonds without formation of by-products. Several compounds are used in the plastics industry:

- acrylic acid, monomer of polyacrylic acid (ion-exchange medium);
- meth(yl)acrylate, monomer of polymethacrylate (plexigum, plastifier);
- methyl methacrylate, monomer of polymethyl methacrylate (perspex = plexiglass, contact lens, dental and orthopedic prostheses, glue); the monomers may be chlorinated;
- acrylonitrile, monomer of polyacrylonitrile (artificial fibre), or as copolymer (*e.g.* with butadiene, styrene, vinyl chloride, vinylidene chloride). Polyacrylonitrile fibres are dissolved in dimethylformamide or dimethylsulfoxide.

Related compounds are acrylamide and methacrylamide, applied as textile finishes, as plastifiers or as copolymers.

Decomposition of the polymers may yield toxic compounds. According to Coleman *et al.* (1954) chlorinated polymethylacrylate disintegrates into HCl and CO. In a non-ventilated department of 100 m^3 a quantity of about $1\frac{1}{2}$ kg resin may present a real hazard in a fire; the irritation caused by HCl, however, serves as warning signal. Oettel (1958) referred to accidental poisoning by acrylonitrile emanating from burning

References p. 168

polyacrylonitrile. According to Underwriters Lab. (1960), burning of Orlon fibres (polyacrylonitrile) yields about the same hazard as the burning of conventional fabrics.

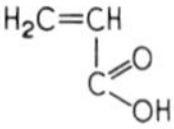
Acrylic acid

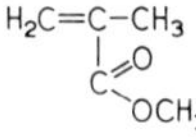
Methyl methacrylate

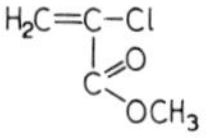
Methyl-α-chloroacrylate

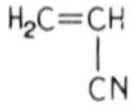
Acrylonitrile

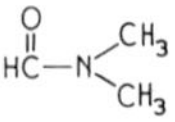
Dimethylformamide

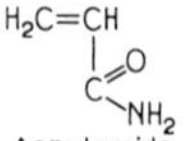
Acrylamide

METHYLACRYLATE, ETHYLACRYLATE

Experimental toxicology and dermatology

Treon *et al.* (1949) and Carpenter *et al.* (1949) reported data on animal toxicity. The minimum oral lethal dose for the rabbit was 0.18–0.28 g/kg for methylacrylate and 0.28–0.42 g/kg for ethylacrylate. The animals became dyspnoeic, convulsive and hypothermic, with severe irritation of digestive tract, degeneration of heart, liver and kidney. Repeated oral intake did not cause cumulative effects. The saturated related compounds (propionates) were much less toxic. Chronic inhalation of 31 p.p.m. for 185 days (7 h per day, 5 days per week) or 95 p.p.m. for 70 days was tolerated without undue effects by rabbits, guinea pigs, rats and monkeys; exposure to concentrations above 200 p.p.m. however was lethal: pulmonary edema, degeneration of the internal organs. The inhalation toxicity was similar for both compounds. The authors suggested as tentative maximum acceptable concentration in industry 75 p.p.m., but emphasized the necessity of medical supervision. Karpov (1954) also observed functional disturbance in the nervous system; he suggested a much lower MAC-value of 20 p.p.m. methacrylate.

Both acrylates proved to be irritating to the animal's skin

and eyes, particularly methylacrylate. Treon *et al.* (1949) applied methyl- and ethylacrylates on the skin of rabbits over periods of 1 to 2 days. Methylacrylate caused intraepithelial pustules, but ethylacrylate completely destroyed the epidermis and, moreover, caused alterations of the viscera.

Industrial toxicology and dermatology

Maglio (1948) pointed out the penetrating, unpleasant sweetish odour; methylacrylate and ethylacrylate have a very strong smell above 31 p.p.m. and 25 p.p.m. respectively. Irritation of the mucosae is reported by Quooss (1959), in addition to some cases of orthoergic dermatoses.

METHYL-α-CHLOROACRYLATE

Experimental toxicology and dermatology

Harris (1953) determined the relation between inhaled concentration and maximal exposure time in groups of 6 rats each: all animals died from pulmonary edema after 5 h exposure to 200 p.p.m., 9 h exposure to 50 p.p.m. and 30–84 h exposure to 10 p.p.m. Goldblatt (1945) obtained similar results. In chronic inhalation (40–60 p.p.m.) experiments Karpov (1957) also noted in addition to irritation of the respiratory tract, degeneration of parenchymatous organs; chronic exposure to 1–6 p.p.m. caused functional disturbance of the central nervous system. He therefore suggested a MAC of 1 p.p.m. Harris (1953) exposed volunteers during a short time to different concentrations with the following results: 250 p.p.m. caused a burning irritation in eyes and headache; 50 p.p.m. flow of tears after 10 sec; 10 p.p.m. and 5 p.p.m. very slight irritation of mucosae after 20 sec. Application of 2 drops to the skin for 20 sec and subsequent washing for 5 min still caused blisters. In animal experiments skin burns and chemical conjunctivitis occurred after application of α-chloroacrylic acid (5 % in water) (Harris 1959); neutralizing with NaOH prevented this effect.

References p. 168

Industrial toxicology and dermatology

Exposure chiefly causes damage to skin or mucosae. The irritative properties warn against inhalation. Harris (1953) reported two cases of skin burns by direct contact; the compound even penetrated rubber. Potassium permanganate is recommended as antidote. Exposure to 5–10 p.p.m. caused photophobia and lachrymation and in the end conjunctivitis. Eyes should be irrigated as soon as possible with 0.65% NaCl (Ridley 1948) after exposure to vapours. In spite of irrigation, a case of corneal ulcer was observed. In 34 workers, exposed for at least a few months to low concentrations of methyl-α-chloroacrylate, no eye diseases were established, but in 19 workers in a production department 5 cases of keratitis punctata were noted. Irritation of air passages did not occur. Karpov (1957) however referred to acute rhinitis, tracheobronchitis, conjunctivitis and headache in workers in such departments.

Skin contact with methyl-α,β-dichloropropionate also caused blisters, because this compound decomposed into methyl-α-chloroacrylate and HCl (Harris 1953). Quooss (1959) also stressed the occurrence of severe keratitis and dermatitis after exposure to α,β-dichloropropionic esters; the effects were noted after a latency time of a few hours, in which the above-mentioned disintegration could take place.

Machining of the polymer polymethyl chloroacrylate (similar to perspex) caused emanation of monomers, resulting in odour and eye troubles (Harris 1953).

METHYL METHACRYLATE, METHYL ETHYLACRYLATE, ETHYL METHACRYLATE, *n*-BUTYL METHACRYLATE

Experimental toxicology and dermatology

Deichmann (1941, 1948) made extensive investigations into the toxicity of methyl methacrylate. The oral LD_{50} for rats was 8.4 ml/kg; the oral MLD for rabbits 7 ml/kg; percutaneous resorption of 10 ml/kg in rabbits caused reversible malaise. Inhalation of 4750 p.p.m. was lethal for rats, guinea pigs and rabbits (depression of respiration, incontinence). Hemoglobinuria was observed in rats and porphyrinuria in rabbits. The compound was corrosive for mucosae and caused local erythema on rabbit skin. Ethyl methacrylate and *n*-butyl methacrylate were less toxic and less volatile than methyl methacrylate. Spealman *et al.* (1945) particularly investigated the chronic toxicity. Exposure of guinea pigs to 9750 p.p.m. 3 h per day for 15 days caused irritation of the respiratory tract; dogs tolerated 10,300 p.p.m. $\frac{1}{2}$ h per day for 15 days but died after exposure to 11,700 p.p.m. $1\frac{1}{2}$ h per day for 8 days (degeneration of liver and kidney). In mice the toxicity of methyl methacrylate was higher than that of acetone, but lower than the toxicity of ethyl acetate. Local application in rabbit eyes caused a reversible chemical conjunctivitis. Filatova (1962) examined rats continuously exposed to methyl methacrylate; she established an amount of 0.1 mg/m^3 as the maximum level below which no reaction of the nervous system occurred. This value should be the MAC.

Spealman *et al.* (1945) performed a prophetic patch test with monomethyl-methacrylate in volunteers: a 48-h patch test showed in one third of 50 students a slight local irritation, but retesting after 10 days proved 10 subjects to be sensitized. Patch tests with plexiglass were negative, also in the sensitized subjects. Nyquist (1958) also sensitized 9 of 20 volunteers by a 48-h patch test with 5% monomer liquid as used in the production of dental prostheses (other agents were therefore also present in this liquid, see below).

Industrial toxicology and dermatology

Workers exposed to fine polymethyl methacrylate dust complained of irritation of the respiratory tract (Queries 1946). According to Harris (1953) the polymer powder also possessed allergic properties, similar to the monomer; he suggested a rather high MAC value of 1000 p.p.m. Machining of plexiglass

References p. 168

(drilling, planing) gives rise to sweetish vapours containing monomers, if local cooling is not applied (Ehrlicher 1962). Karpov (1953, 1954) observed irritability, tiredness, drowsiness, headache, anorexia, hypotension in workers exposed to monomer vapours. Irritation of the mucosae occurred at 62 p.p.m. He suggested therefore a much lower MAC value of 12.5 p.p.m. (= 50 mg/m^3). Rajnes (1957) found even this value too high, because at exposures to 12.5–25 p.p.m. for 20–90 min dizziness, drowsiness, sickness and loss of consciousness were reported. Sandratzkaya (1961) examined 80 workers, mostly female, in a button factory; they were exposed to maximal 800–950 mg methyl methacrylate/m^3. She reported an increased incidence of hypotonia, atrophic rhinitis, conjunctivitis and general neurovegetative disorders. Blood and urine were normal.

Elkins (1959) suggested a MAC value of 100 p.p.m. (= 400 mg/m^3).

Reports on skin manifestations due to acrylic compounds mainly concern their uses in the manufacture and repair of dental prostheses in which intimate skin contact is unavoidable.

The ingredients used on an industrial scale do not differ largely from those used in dental prostheses (Malten 1956), and therefore the following data may be useful in the scope of this work. The greatest skin risks occur during the cold-curing process in which two-compound mixtures are used containing the following ingredients (Malten 1960, Kleine-Natrop 1960):

1. *Monomer liquid* may contain:
   a. methyl methacrylate
      methacrylic acid anhydride, vinyl methacrylate } used in copolymerization to form three-dimensional net structures.
   b. radical donor: benzoyl peroxide (in surplus)
   c. inhibitor: hydroquinone, resorcin, phenol, pyrogallol, pyridine, benzoic acid, eugenol, thymol, etc.

d. plasticizer: dibutyl phthalate, triphenyl phosphate, glycol, fatty acid alcohols, paladinol, etc.
e. solvent: trichloroethylene, methylene chloride, ethylene chloride, chloroform, etc.

2. *Polymer powder* may contain:
   a. polymethyl methacrylate (medium molecular)
   b. catalyst: dimethyl *p*-toluidine, aliphatic amines, mercaptanes, sulfinic acids, hydrazine compounds, etc.
   c. pigments of various origin.

Mixing of catalyst with radical donor results in the formation of radicals. These react with the double bonds of the monomers to give rise to the formation of radical monomers, thus starting the chain-propagation reaction, which leads to the final macromolecular product. According to Axelsson (1955) the end-product still may contain 3 to 5% of 'rest monomer', containing some real monomer, some di- to penta-mer, and for the greater part low-molecular polymer. (This, presumably, is due to the necessity of using a surplus of radical donor for the starting reaction, which promotes the formation of many reaction centres and thus the formation of relatively short chains). According to Spealman *et al.* (1945) monomeric methyl methacrylate has to be considered as a sensitizer. Werner (1958) has demonstrated the occurrence of sensitization to intermediate methyl methacrylate products in patients not reacting to monomethyl methacrylate or the polymethacrylic end-product (he did not exclude possible sensitization to auxiliary substances). Fisher (1954) considered heat-cured methacrylates as being totally inert, and Patty (1949) was of opinion that only stabilizers and antioxidants might have adverse physiological effects, particularly dermatitis. Benzoyl peroxide has been cited as a sensitizing agent in the flour industry (Grosfeld 1951) and in processing unsaturated polyester resins (Malten 1956) (see Chapters 7 and 16). On the other hand, Harris (1959) is of the opinion that sawing of plexiglass may set free unreacted methacrylate monomer; skin contact with the sawdust can cause contact eczema situated on the back of the hands and in the interdigital spaces (which is a typical localization for a dust dissolved in sweat). During a 7-year observation in the Fokker aircraft works where plexiglass windows were glued in metal frames and where astralon plates (copolymer of vinyl chloride with methyl methacrylate) were used for the construction of refrigerators, Malten only once observed a contact sensitization to methyl methacrylate monomer of questionable origin. Bouffioux (1959) described a case with general manifestations, an urticarial exanthema and positive patch tests occurring 7 years after implantation of an acrylic femurcup prosthesis.

ACRYLAMIDE AND METHACRYLAMIDE

Stokinger (1956) reported the toxicological properties of acrylamide, as established in animal experiments. The acute oral toxicity is relatively low, but after chronic uptake a considerable neurotoxicity is present: ataxia, tremor of the hind legs, muscle atrophy. The chronic neurotoxic effect is reversible, but a recurrence takes place after a relatively low uptake. The effects do not increase in intensity with larger doses. Oettel (1958) observed signs similar to multiple sclerosis in all species of animals after repeated uptake of 50 mg acrylamide/kg/day or 100 mg methacrylamide/kg/day. Daily sub-toxic doses for one year, however, did not give rise to neurologic symptoms: cumulative effects did not occur. According to Oettel, symptoms in workers in industry had not been reported, because the compounds were not penetrating through the skin. The American Cyanamid Corp. (undated), however, published data about the toxicity of berylamide (acrylamide), pointing to the possibility of percutaneous resorption. The compound in 1% solution proved also to be irritating to human skin.

ACRYLONITRILE

Experimental toxicology and dermatology

The acute and chronic toxicity was studied systematically by Dudley *et al.* (1942a, 1942b). Species sensitivity was obvious: dogs became poisoned by 65 p.p.m. for 4 h, whereas monkeys tolerated 90 p.p.m. with only minor effects; guinea pigs particularly tolerated high dosage. The acute symptoms were similar to those of experimental HCN poisoning: hyperpnoea (followed by slow and shallow breathing), convulsions, coma, death; the peripheral parts of the body became red. The guinea pigs only showed other symptoms: pulmonary edema. Administration of $NaNO_2$ had an antidotal effect (not in guinea pigs). Chronic inhalation of 60 p.p.m. 4 h per day, 5 days per week for 4 weeks caused a serious intoxication in dogs, but not in other species. Cumulative effects were not present. On autopsy a slight hemosiderosis, interstitial nephritis and bronchopneumonia was seen. The toxic dose of acrylonitrile calculated per quantity –CN corresponded very well with the toxicity of HCN. Dudley *et al.* therefore proposed a MAC of 20 p.p.m. Smyth *et al.* (1948) established the same order of toxicity as Dudley *et al.*; they also proved the possibility of percutaneous resorption (LD_{50} for rabbits 0.25 g/kg). A slight degeneration of the liver in dogs (30–40 p.p.m. $6\frac{1}{2}$ h per day, 5 days per week, 10 weeks) was noted by Wilson *et al.* (1948). Brieger *et al.* (1952) also established the greater sensitivity of dogs; they explained the relative tolerance to acrylonitrile in rats as opposed to dogs by the better detoxication into thiocyanates in the former. However, according to Benes *et al.* (1959) the symptoms of poisoning in rats are not primarily caused by –CN, but chiefly by the acrylonitrile molecule itself. These authors established once more the antidotal effects of the usual –CN antiodotes $NaNO_2$ and Na-thiosulphate. Magos (1962) also found that CN-metabolite formation in rats killed by acrylonitrile is much lower than in animals killed by KCN; in rats, therefore,

References p. 168

the toxicity of acrylonitrile could not be solely due to liberation of –CN. Magos also pointed out the great species specificity.

The animal experiments offer strong arguments in discriminating the –CN ion as the chief toxic agent in acrylonitrile poisoning (except in guinea pigs): similarity of clinical symptoms; equivalence of toxic doses; increase of thiocyanate excretion and of –CN and CN-metabolic levels in blood; antidotal effects of $NaNO_2$ and Na-thiosulphate; presence of almond odour.

The biological effects of polyacrylonitrile dust (percentage of monomer $< 0.1\%$) in rabbits were investigated by Massmann (1956a). Intratracheal injection (24 mg in 1.5 ml aq., diam. $< 5\mu$) did not cause fibrosis; purulent pneumonia and reversible granulomata, however, did occur. Systemic poisoning was not present. Lomonova (1962), however, reported serious toxic effects in rats exposed to 1.3 mg polyacrylonitrile/m^3 (1 h per day, 45 days): rhinorrhea, progressive albuminuria, monocytosis, degeneration of liver and kidney, parenchymatous hyperplasia of the thyroid. The practical consequences of this observation for industry are not clear, because the concentration in air was excessively high.

Industrial toxicology and dermatology

Wilson *et al.* (1944, 1948) examined workers in a rubber factory: production of copolymerizates from butadiene, styrene and acrylonitrile. The last compound proved to be the most toxic. Exposure to 16–100 p.p.m. for 20–45 min caused symptoms: headache, oppression, irritation of air passages, apprehension, irritability, itching skin; sometimes also sickness, vomiting, headache, asthenia and diarrhoea was noted. One case of serious hepatic disease and several cases of slight jaundice (with painful liver) were observed, mostly with slight anemia and leucocytosis. The thiocyanate concentration in the blood returned to normal levels when the subjects were exposed to < 22 p.p.m. for 30 min, but at exposure above 50 p.p.m. the level did not reach normal values within 12 h. According to Mallette (1943) an uptake of the toxic agent is proved, if in non-smokers the thiocyanate level in serum exceeds 2 mg/100 ml and the concentration in urine 2 mg/l (in smokers 3 mg/100 ml and 16 mg/l respectively). Djuric *et al.* (1962) gave 30 mg/h as discriminating level in smokers. Brieger *et al.* (1952) however very strongly doubted the practical value of this biological test, because of the large normal variation and the strong influence of smoking. According to Hofmann (1961) exposure to 20 p.p.m. causes irritation of mucosa, headache, nervous instability.

Some non-industrial lethal poisonings in children by acrylonitrile used as insecticide (Ventox), rubbed into the hair, were reported by Grumske (1949) and Lorz (1950); the clinical symptoms were similar to HCN poisoning.

Dudley *et al.* (1942a) and Wilson *et al.* (1948) pointed out the severe orthoergic effects on the skin: direct contact caused blisters, desquamation and slow healing. While he doubted the occurrence of systemic intoxication in industry, Aubertin (1960) stressed the hazard of skin diseases: erythema with vesicles, sometimes with a latency period of 24 h. In 1954, Wilson *et al.* stressed again that skin contact should be avoided, not only because of the vesicant action, but also because of possible toxic systemic effects: immediate washing with copious quantities of soap and water is considered necessary. Acrylonitrile may cause contact dermatitis (*Hygienic Guide*, series 1957); one is left to guess what is meant by this statement.

DIMETHYLFORMAMIDE, DIMETHYLSULFOXIDE

Experimental toxicology and dermatology

Massmann (1956b) established the toxicity of dimethylformamide in mice, rats, rabbits and cats. The LD_{50} (oral) for rats was 0.14–0.38 ml/100 g. Inhalation of 420 p.p.m., 8 h/day, 6 days per week for 120 days did not give rise to toxic effects in rats. The compound is absorbed percutaneously; damage of liver and kidney were the most important pathological effects. Lobanova (1958) not only observed degeneration of parenchym-

References p. 168

atous organs, but also disturbance of higher nervous activity and microscopical changes in the interneuronal system. These effects were noted in rats exposed to 100–160 p.p.m., 4 h/day for 6 months; exposure to 10–16 p.p.m. did not give rise to toxic effects. Lobanova therefore suggested a MAC value of 15 p.p.m. (= 50 mg/m^3); because of the low volatility she estimated the industrial hazard to be rather low. Another Russian author (Odosasvili 1962), however, came in similar experiments to a much lower MAC value: 0.03 mg/m^3. Martelli (1960) observed lethal effects in guinea pigs after percutaneous resorption (10 ml/day for 7–9 days on shaven skin); degeneration of liver and kidney were present. The toxicity in mice was determined by Fugisaki (1960); percutaneous uptake was also proved in these animals. Only Hofmann (1961) did not observe any liver disease in rats and cats; even exposure of cats to 1000 p.p.m., 6 h/day for 10 weeks or to 300 p.p.m. for 15 months did not cause any functional or anatomical liver degeneration. He denied therefore the specific liver toxicity of dimethylformamide and judged the proposed MAC value of 20 p.p.m. too low.

From experiments on mice and rabbits Uramuna (1960) concluded that dimethylsulfoxide was one of the least toxic solvents, although inhalation of high concentrations might be hazardous (LD_{50} subc. inj. 25–64 mg/g in mice).

Industrial toxicology and dermatology

In a period of 15 months, Tolot *et al.* (1958) observed in 11 workers (total exposed numbers not reported) rather serious disturbances of health. Although the subjects were exposed to dimethylformamide, cyclohexanol, $SnCl_2$ and oxalic acid, the authors incriminated the first compound because of the occupational history. After exposure for a few weeks to some months, the following complaints were noted:

– Symptoms from the digestive tract were preponderant (sickness, vomiting, burning pain in esophageal and gastric area; stomach ulcers were not observed).

– General vegetative symptoms (anorexia, disturbance of sleep, sensitivity to alcohol).
– Itching skin, sometimes dermatoses.
– In two cases a liver disease was observed.

Symptoms in the respiratory tract and blood dyscrasia did not occur. The authors warned against the employment of workers with gastric disorders or liver diseases (*cave*: alcoholics). Commencing skin disease healed very quickly if the hands were immersed in acid solution (acetic acid or formic acid 5 %). Martelli (1960) also reported the occurrence of liver diseases; he warned against skin contact. A MAC value of 50 p.p.m. = 150 mg/m³ was suggested.

SPECIFIC PREVENTION

Excessive inhalation of the above-mentioned compounds should be prevented. The MAC values recommended by A.C.G.I.H. (1962) may serve as a guide to ventilation engineers; if possible, the concentration levels should be below these values, as several authors suggest lower levels. The relevant American values, as given in 1962, are:

acrylonitrile	20 p.p.m.	=	45 mg/m³
dimethylformamide	20 p.p.m.	=	60 mg/m³
ethylacrylate	25 p.p.m.	=	100 mg/m³
methylacrylate	10 p.p.m.	=	35 mg/m³

Other less generally accepted values, have already been mentioned.

The value of 20 p.p.m. for acrylonitrile seems to be rather high in regard to the reported industrial experiences; the Russian value of 0.25 p.p.m. = 0.5 mg/m³ (Nesswetha 1960), on the other hand, seems to be extraordinarily low.

Because of the orthoergic or allergic properties of many compounds, and because of the possibility of percutaneous resorption of some of these, skin contact should be prevented as much as possible. Rubber gloves do not always protect sufficiently.

REFERENCES

American Conference Governmental Industrial Hygienists, *Threshold Limit Values*, Detroit, Michigan, 1962.

American Cyanamid Corporation, *Berylamide*, Technical bulletin, Petrochem. Dept., New York.

Aubertin, X., Intoxications par l'acide cyanhydrique et ses dérivés; leur thérapeutique d'urgence. *Arch. Maladies Prof.*, 21 (1960) 643.

Axelsson, B., Degree of polymerization of methylmethacrylate in relation to curing time and temperature. *Odontol. Rev.*, 6 (1955) 124.

Benes, V. and C. Cerna, Acute toxicity and action of acrylonitrile. *J. Hyg. Epidemiol. Microbiol. Immunol. (Prague)*, 3 (1959) 106. Ref.: *Bull. Hyg.*, 34 (1959) 791.

Bouffioux, J., Allergie à l'acrylique, manifestations cutanées et générales. *Arch. Belges Dermatol.*, 15 (1959) 336.

Brieger, H., F. Rieders and W. A. Hodes, Acrylonitrile: spectrophotometric determination, acute toxicity and mechanism of action. *Arch. Ind. Hyg.*, 6 (1952) 128.

Carpenter, C. P., H. F. Smyth and U. C. Pozzani, The assay of acute vapor toxicity and the grading and interpretation of results on 96 chemical compounds. *J. Ind. Hyg.*, 31 (1949) 343.

Coleman, E. H. and C. H. Thomas, The products of combustion of chlorinated plastics. *J. Appl. Chem.*, 4 (1954) 379.

Deichmann, W. B., Toxicity of methyl, ethyl and butyl methacrylate. *J. Ind. Hyg.*, 23 (1941) 343.

Deichmann, W. B. and E. G. Mergard, Comparative evaluation of methods employed to express degree of toxicity of compound. *J. Ind. Hyg.*, 30 (1948) 373.

Djuric, D., P. Raicevic and I. Konstantinovic, Excretion of thiocyanates in urine of smokers. *Arch. Environ. Health*, 5 (1962) 18.

Dudley, H. C. and P. A. Neal, Toxicology of acrylonitrile. I. A study of acute toxicity. *J. Ind. Hyg.*, 24 (1942a) 27.

Dudley, H. C., T. R. Sweeney and J. W. Miller, Toxicology of acrylonitrile. II. Studies of effects of daily inhalation. *J. Ind. Hyg.*, 24 (1942b) 255.

Ehrlicher, H., Arbeitsmedizinische Fragen auf den Kunststoffgebiet. *Kongress f. Arbeitsschutz 1961*, Steinkopf, Darmstadt, 1962.

ELKINS, H. B., *The Chemistry of Industrial Toxicology*, 2nd ed., Wiley, New York; Chapman & Hall, London, 1959.

FILATOVA, V. I., Data for substantiating the maximum permissible concentration of methyl methacrylate in the atmospheric air. *Gig. Sanitaria*, 27, 11 (1962) 3.

FISHER, A. A., Allergic sensitization of the skin and oral mucosa to acrylic denture materials. *J. Am. Med. Assoc.*, 156 (1954) 238.

FUGISAKI, K., A study on the toxicity of dimethylformamide as a solvent. *Igaku Kenkyu*, 30 (1960) 2291. Ref.: *Bull. Hyg.*, 36 (1961) 535.

GOLDBLATT, M. W., Vesication and some vesicants. *Brit. J. Ind. Med.*, 2 (1945) 183.

GROSFELD, J. C. M., *Onderzoekingen over het ontstaan van eczeem bij bakkers*, Thesis, Amsterdam, 1951.

GRUMSKE, T., Ventox und Ventox Vergiftung. *Deut. Med. Wochschr.*, 74 (1949) 1081.

HARRIS, D. K., Health problems in the manufacture and use of plastics. *Brit. J. Ind. Med.*, 10 (1953) 255.

HARRIS, D. K., Some hazards in the manufacture and use of plastics. *Brit. J. Ind. Med.*, 16 (1959) 221.

HOFMANN, H. T., Zur Frage der Gesundheitsgefährdung durch moderne Kunststoffe und ihre Lösungsmittel. *Zbl. Arbeitsmed.*, 11 (1961) 240.

Hygienic Guide, Acrylonitrile. *Am. Ind. Hyg. Assoc. Quart.*, 18 (1957) 78.

KARPOV, B. D., Effect of small concentrations of methyl methacrylate vapors on the inhibition and stimulation processes of the cortex of the brain. *Trans. Leningrad Sanit. Gig. Med. Inst.*, 14 (1953) 43. Ref.: WILSON *et al.*, 1960.

KARPOV, B. D., Methyl methacrylate from the viewpoint of labor hygiene. *Gigiena i Sanit.*, 19 (1954) 25. Ref.: WILSON *et al.*, 1960.

KARPOV, B. D., Toxicity of methyl acrylate. *Farmakol. i Toksikol.*, 17 (1954) 49. Ref.: *Arch. Ind. Health*, 12 (1955) 665.

KARPOV, B. D., Angaben zur toxikologischen Charakteristik von Methylchlorakrylat. *Gigiena i Sanit.*, 22/4 (1957) 74. Ref.: *Zbl. Arbeitsmed.*, 9 (1959) 275.

KLAUDER, J. V., Patch-test study to determine cutaneous reactions to new compounds. *Arch. Environ. Health*, 1 (1960) 407.

KLEINE-NATROP, H. E., Berufsbedingte Paladon-ekzeme bei Zahntechnikern. *Berufsdermatosen*, 8 (1960) 301.

LOBANOVA, K. P., Toxicity of dimethylformamide. *Gigiena i Sanit.*, 23, 5 (1958) 31.

LOMONOVA, G. V., Toxicological characteristics of the acrylonitrile polymer. *Gigiena Truda i Prof. Zabolevaniya*, 6/6 (1962) 54.

LORZ, H., Über perkutane Vergiftung mit Akrylnitril (Ventox). *Deut. Med. Wochschr.*, 75 (1950) 1087.

MAGLIO, M. M., Identification of acrylate and methacrylate polymer and copolymer resins. *Chemist-Analyst*, 37 (1948) 4. Ref.: TREON *et al.*, 1949.

MAGOS, L., A study of acrylonitrile poisoning in relation to methaemoglobin–CN complex formation, *Brit. J. Ind. Med.*, 19 (1962) 283.

MALLETTE, F. S., Industrial hygiene in synthetic rubber manufacture. *Ind. Med.*, 12 (1943) 495.

MALTEN, K. E., *Beroepseczeem bij het verwerken van kunststoffen*, Thesis, Amsterdam, 1956.

MALTEN, K. E., Allergische reacties op kunstharsen. *Tijdschr. Tandheelk.*, 67 (1960) 827.

MARTELLI, D., Toxicology of dimethylformamide. *Med. Lavoro*, 51 (1960) 123. Ref.: *Bull. Hyg.*, 35 (1960) 972.

MASSMANN, W., Untersuchungen über die biologische Wirkung des Polyacrylnitrils. *Z. Ges. Exptl. Med.*, 127 (1956a) 409.

MASSMANN, W., Toxicological investigations on di-methylformamide. *Brit. J. Ind. Med.*, 13 (1956b) 51.

NESSWETHA, W., Über die maximalen Arbeitsplatzkonzentrationen in der USSR. *Zbl. Arbeitsmed.*, 10 (1960) 112.

NYQUIST, G., Sensitivity to methyl methacrylate. *Trans. Roy. Schools Dentistry (Stockholm)*, 1 (1958) 35.

ODOSASVILI, D. G., Determining the MAC of dimethyl-formamide in the atmosphere. *Gig. Sanitaria*, 27, 4 (1962) 3.

OETTEL, H., Gesundheitsgefährdung durch Kunststoffe? *Naunyn-Schmiedeberg's Arch. Exptl. Pathol. Pharmakol.*, 232 (1958) 77.

PATTY, F. A., *Industrial Hygiene and Toxicology*, Vol. II, Interscience, New York, 1949.

Queries and Minor Notes, Toxicity of plexiglass. *J. Am. Med. Assoc.*, 131 (1946) 1103.

QUOOSS, H., *Gesundheitsgefahren in der Kunststoffindustrie*, Barth, Leipzig, 1959.

RAJNES, L. A., Angaben zur Charakteristik der Toxizität von Methylmethakrylat unter den Arbeitsbedingungen einer Fabrik für zahnärztlichen Beruf. *Gigiena Truda i Prof. Zabolevaniya*, 1 (1957) 56. Ref.: *Zbl. Arbeitsmed.*, 9 (1959) 275.

RIDLEY, F., The use and abuse of topical ocular therapy. *Trans. Ophthalmol. Soc. U.K.*, 68 (1948) 301. Ref.: HARRIS, 1953.

SANDRATZKAJA, S. E., Polymethyl-methacrylate. *Gigiena i Sanit.*, 7 (1961) 74.

SMYTH, H. F. and C. P. CARPENTER, Further experience with the range finding test in the industrial toxicology laboratory. *J. Ind. Hyg.*, 30 (1948) 63.

SPEALMAN, C. R., R. J. MAIN, H. B. HAAG and P. S. LARSON, Monomeric methyl methacrylate; studies on toxicity. *Ind. Med. Surg.*, 14 (1945) 292.

STOKINGER, H. E., Advances in industrial toxicology for the year 1955. *Arch. Ind. Health*, 14 (1956) 206.

TOLOT, F., M. DROIN and GENEVOIS, Intoxication par la diméthylformamide. *Arch. Maladies Prof.*, 19 (1958) 602.

TREON, J. F., H. SIGMON, H. WRIGHT and K. V. KITZMILLER, The toxicity of methyl and ethyl acrylate. *J. Ind. Hyg.*, 31 (1949) 317.

Underwriter's Laboratories, *Miscellaneous hazard*, 5148. Oct. 1960. Ref.: ZAPP, 1962.

URAMUNA, T., An experimental study of the toxicity of dimethylsulfoxide as a solvent. *Igaku Kenkyu*, 30 (1960) 2235. Ref.: *Bull. Hyg.*, 36 (1961) 535.

WERNER, M., Zur Diagnostik der Paladon-Allergie. *Allergie u. Asthma*, 4 (1958) 1.

WILSON, R. H., Health hazards encountered in the manufacture of synthetic rubber. *J. Am. Med. Assoc.*, 124 (1944) 701.

WILSON, R. H., G. V. HOUGH and W. E. MCCORMICK, Medical problems encountered in the manufacture of American-made rubber. *Ind. Med. Surg.*, 17 (1948) 199.

WILSON, R. H. and W. E. MCCORMICK, Acrylonitrile: its physiology and toxicology. *Ind. Med. Surg.*, 18 (1949) 243.

WILSON, R. H. and W. E. MCCORMICK, Toxicology of plastics and rubber plastomers and monomers. *Ind. Med. Surg.*, 23 (1954) 479.

WILSON, R. H. and W. E. MCCORMICK, Plastics: the toxicology of synthetic resins. *Arch. Ind. Health*, 21 (1960) 536.

ZAPP, J. A., Toxic and health effects of plastics and resins. *Arch. Environ. Health*, 4 (1962) 335.

12

Fluorine-containing polymers

PHYSICO-CHEMICAL PROPERTIES, APPLICATION

The following polymers are included in this group:
- polytetrafluoroethylene: $[CF_2CF_2]_n$ (Teflon, Fluon)
- polymonochlorotrifluoroethylene: $[CClFCF_2]_n$ (Kel-F, Fluorothen, Hostaflon)
- polyvinyl fluoride: $[CH_2CHF]_n$
- copolymers, *e.g.:* fluoroelastomers.

These polymers are chemically highly inert substances, possessing valuable mechanical and electrical properties. The cost still restricts their wide application. Generally, the fluorine-containing polymers are used as thermoplastics; the resins may be machined (fraising, planing, sawing, boring). For surface-coating, the spraying of a dispersion in 10% chromic acid is applied; the coating has to be heated to 400° (I.C.I. 1959).

PRODUCTS OF DECOMPOSITION

Because of its hygienic significance, the process of decomposition must be dealt with in greater detail. Several investigators have tried to measure (semi-)quantitatively the products of decomposition by different methods. In the following schematic review particulars of the methods used had to be omitted.

Temperature below 150°: no decomposition.

Temperature 150–200°: according to information supplied

by the French army and airforce authorities (1958), formation of HF may occur at 180°. This is not in accordance with most investigations.

Temperature 200–250°: Dupont de Nemours (undated) mentioned a slight decomposition into toxic products at 204–316°. Gancberg (1959) did not find any decomposition after heating a silicon–Teflon mixture for 32 h at 200°, or for 9 h at 250° and subsequently for 22 h at 300°.

Temperature 250–300°: according to I.C.I. (1959b) the decomposition of Fluon starts in a minor degree at 250–300°. Sendroy *et al.* (1952) heated an engine of a submarine, insulated with polytetrafluoroethylene: they determined CO and HF in the surrounding air. The concentration of CO did not exceed the MAC value; the results regarding HF were inconclusive. At 260° Teflon decreases in weight by 0.0001 to 0.0006‰, depending on the type of polymer (Zapp 1962).

Temperature 300–350°: Dupont de Nemours (undated) reported on a continuous heating of Teflon at 316° for 14 months. The decrease in weight was less than 1‰; 1 kg Teflon heated for 1 h at 316° produced 0.6 ml gaseous products. Many other plastics showed a much higher decrease of weight. According to Madorsky *et al.* (1953) and Troyanowsky (1959), pyrolysis of polytetrafluoroethylene below 335° did not produce any decomposition products; Zapp *et al.* (1955), however, mentioned the occurrence of hexafluoroethane at 300–360°.

Temperature 350–400°: in contrast to most authors Dehez (1957) denied any decomposition of Teflon below 400°. The producer of Fluon (I.C.I. 1959b), however, mentioned the possibility of poisoning by decomposition products (mixture of FC components with traces of HF) after heating to 350°. Zapp *et al.* (1955, 1962) established the presence of octofluoroisobutylene at temperatures of 380° and higher. Gancberg (1959) heated spiral Teflon foils for 10 h and hardly saw any decomposition below 400°.

Temperature 400–450°: Madorsky *et al.* (1953) pyrolysed

References p. 180

polytetrafluoroethylene between 423 and 513°, and saw a complete decomposition into the monomer C_2F_4. A quick heating of Teflon (coated on copper wire) up to above 400° produced a complete destruction of the polymer with possible formation of octofluoroisobutylene and oxygen difluoride (Treon *et al.* 1955). Heating up to 390–445° caused an increase of weight because of oxidation, heating above 445° caused a decrease, the rate increasing quickly above 500° (Troyanowsky 1959). According to Dupont de Nemours (undated) the concentration of F_2 (→HF) in the gaseous products above 400° never exceeded 0.5%; Troyanowsky however reported higher concentrations.

Temperature 450–500°: above 445° Troyanowsky (1959) determined the following products of decomposition: tetrafluoroethylene, hexafluoropropene, octofluorocyclobutane, and at the most very small quantities of octofluoroisobutylene.

Temperature 500–550°: Zapp *et al.* (1955) established the following products of decomposition: tetrafluoroethylene, hexafluoropropylene, octofluorocyclobutane, octofluoroisobutylene and perfluoro-olefines. Siegle *et al.* (1956) found after pyrolysis *in vacuo* at 510°: 97.2% tetrafluoroethylene, 2.65% hexafluoropropylene, 0.1% tetrafluoromethane.

Temperature 550° and above: Atkinson *et al.* (1953) heated gaseous monomer tetrafluoroethylene: at about 550° they found octofluorocyclobutane, at 600–700° hexafluoropropylene and octofluoroisobutylene and above 800° free radicals as a source of hexafluoroethane and polymerized unsaturated products.

Some notes have to added to the above-mentioned data:

– The investigators used widely different experimental procedures; nevertheless, the resultant data showed reasonable correspondence.

– The products of decomposition consist of gas and of a sublimate of solid compounds.

– Impure Teflon (*e.g.* Teflon enamels, mixtures with minerals) are reported to have lower temperatures of decomposition (Troyanowsky 1959). The recent types are more pure than older

ones; lethal temperature for rats therefore lies higher (Zapp 1962).
– The chlorinated product Kel-F decomposes at lower temperatures than Teflon (Treon *et al.* 1955, Dehez 1957).
– It should be emphasized that many other plastics have a higher rate of decomposition than the fluorine-containing polymers, also with production of toxic substances.

From these results, the following conclusions may be drawn regarding the decomposition of F-containing polymers:
– The quality and quantity of the products are chiefly determined by the temperature.
– At 250–300° decomposition starts; above 350–400° the rate of this process increases.
– The decomposition products are: the monomer (C_2F_4), ($F_2 \rightarrow HF$), aliphatic and cyclic saturated and unsaturated CF compounds.

EXPERIMENTAL TOXICOLOGY

Polymers

These compounds are chemically inert and therefore also biologically inactive. In animal experiments ingestion and inhalation did not produce any pathological effects (Zapp *et al.* 1955).

Products of decomposition

Many investigators have examined the toxicity of these compounds, alerted by the unfavorable experiences in industry. Frodsham (1951) exposed groups of two rats each to vapours emanating from decomposition of Fluon under the following conditions:

140–150° for 3–5 h caused slight irritation of air passages; 260° for $\frac{1}{2}$ h caused manifest irritation; 300° for 2 h resulted in pulmonary edema; 315° for 1 h and subsequently 315–325° for $\frac{1}{2}$ h the following day caused depression and pulmonary edema.

A group of 6 rats was exposed by Sendroy *et al.* (1952) in an unventilated room to vapours emanating from a submarine

References p. 180

engine isolated with polytetrafluoroethylene; the temperature of the engine was 150, 200, 250 or 300° (burn-out) in different experiments. The rats did not exhibit any pathological effects. Hagemeyer *et al.* (1954) exposed groups of mice to decomposition products of polytetrafluoroethylene; if the concentration of halogens in the air did not exceed 10 p.p.m., no effect was observed; at 100 p.p.m. some of the mice died, at 1000 p.p.m. all died within 30 seconds. According to Treon *et al.* (1954, 1955) the mortality of animals was roughly parallel to the quantity of Teflon decomposed at temperatures above 400°. Guinea pigs, mice, rats and rabbits were more sensitive than cats and dogs. The toxicity of the decomposition products was not enhanced by raising the temperature from 500 to 800°, but at lower temperatures the products were much less toxic. At 800°, the presence of O_2 enhanced the toxicity if small quantities of Teflon were decomposed. The toxicity of Kel-F and Teflon regarding decomposition was in the same order of magnitude. Treon *et al.* described the following effects: chemical pneumonitis, diffuse degeneration of liver, kidney and brain, bloody discharge from the nostrils, dyspnoea, convulsions, etching of the cornea.

Zapp *et al.* (1955) exposed rats for some hours to one of the above-mentioned decomposition products: 0.5 p.p.m. octofluoroisobutylene; the animals died from pulmonary edema. The authors estimated the toxicity as 10 times that of phosgene. Exposure of rats by Harris (1959) for 6 h to decomposition products of Fluon caused no symptoms at 250°, irritation at 275°, lethal pulmonary edema at 300°. Truffert (1959) exposed several species of animals to decomposition (658°) of polytetrafluoroethylene, coated on aluminum sheets, with the following results: 970 mg polymer/m^2 Al (60 min, guinea pigs) slight irritation of passages; 3340 mg/m^2 Al (60 min, guinea pigs) strong irritation; exposure of rabbits, rats and mice for 60 min to 974 mg/m^2 Al, 1023 mg/m^2 Al and 978 mg/m^2 Al respectively resulted in slight irritation in all animals.

These results are not in agreement with those of Treon *et al.*

(1954, 1955), but presumably in the latter case the quantity of decomposition products was much larger.

Cavagna *et al.* (1961) established a pathogenesis of Teflon fume fever similar to zinc fume fever: phagocytosis of the sublimate results in the production of endogenous pyrogens; particles of polymer taken up by leucocytes probably set free these pyrogenous substances (Pernis *et al.* 1961).

Lester *et al.* (1950), Pattison (1959) and Clayton *et al.* (1960) determined the toxicity of possible products of decomposition of several fluorine-containing hydrocarbons. Their data may be summarized as follows:

negligible toxicity: polyfluoroalkanes, 1,1-difluoroethylene, vinylidene fluoride, vinyl fluoride, octofluorocyclobutane;

moderate toxicity: 1,1-dichloro-2,2-difluoroethylene;

high toxicity: tetrafluoroethylene, polyfluoroalkenes, polychlorofluoroalkenes, octofluoroisobutylene (perfluoroisobutylene), hexafluoropropylene (perfluoropropylene), monochlorotrifluoroethylene.

Pattison emphasized the hazard of volatile components with CF_2 groups, as causing pulmonary edema. Attention should be paid to the investigations of Daniskevsky *et al.* (1961), who concluded that the toxic hazard of many fluorine-containing compounds is largely determined by admixture of the very toxic octofluoroisobutylene.

From the above-mentioned data, the following *conclusions* may be drawn:

- heating of polytetrafluoroethylene at 200 to 300° may cause transient slight or moderate irritation of the mucosae of the air passages.
- heating at temperatures above 300° may result in severe irritation, possible pulmonary edema,
- heating at temperatures above 500° may lead to death of animals in short time,
- particularly the unsaturated fluorine-containing compounds may be considered as very toxic decomposition products; these compounds occur above 300 to 400°.

References p. 180

INDUSTRIAL TOXICOLOGY AND DERMATOLOGY

Unfavorable experiences became known as soon as fluorine-containing polymers were processed in industry. In fact, these experiences gave the impetus to much of the above-mentioned experimental work. Already in 1951, Harris had described four industrial cases of a febrile illness, resembling 'metal fume fever'. The workmen developed a feeling of influenza, 'cold', malaria: following an irritation of the air passages, possibly with dry coughing and restrosternal oppression ('tightness'), there were shivers with increase of temperature, pulse and respiratory rate, ultimately with profuse sweating. Physical examination hardly revealed anything, sometimes a few râles; slight leucocytosis was sometimes present. The symptoms were reversible within 24 hours. The workers were exposed to decomposition products of polytetrafluoroethylene at 400–450°. The 'polymer fume fever' described never occurred if the processing temperatures did not exceed 350°. One of the workers, however, developed fever also after exposure to fine cold polymer dust. Sherwood (1955) and Challen *et al.* (1955) described seven cases of a similar illness from a department, where Fluon was heated at 350–380°, and machined afterwards. One of the workers excreted 5 mg fluorine/l urine during an attack. X-ray of the lungs in two cases did not reveal any pathology. One worker suffered from conjunctivitis. Most of the workmen in the department complained of some symptoms at one time or another. At first the concentration of Fluon in air was up to 3.5 mg/m^3; a decrease to 0.2–0.4 mg/m^3 (very small particle size) did not sufficiently reduce the occurrence of symptoms. Of the seven workmen with the above-described symptoms, 6 were smoking during the work, and the non-smoker worked close to an oven. The authors stressed the importance of smoking: decomposition of one particle of Fluon of 1 mm diameter during smoking would correspond to an exposure for 8 h to 0.4 mg Fluon/m^3. Harris (1959) described two further cases of 'polymer fume fever' in workmen, who smoked while processing Fluon. Strict prohibition of smoking seems therefore necessary. Two workmen who sprayed a dispersion in chromic acid developed an irritation of the skin; the acid was probably the offending agent.

A rather alarming statement was issued by the National Advisory Council for Aeronautics in the U.S.A. (1956): decomposition products were said to have caused a fatal illness in one worker. Extensive investigations, however, conclusively disproved this: the information was 'definitely not true' (Dupont de Nemours, undated), a 'complete lie' (I.C.I., 1959 b).

The industrial experiences reported here indicate an occurrence of 'polymer fume fever' after exposure to decomposition products of fluorine-containing polymers. Temporary immunity as in Zn-fever does not seem to establish itself. As a rule, complete recovery sets in within 24 h, no after-effects are known. Smoking seems to be an important factor; probably not the exposure to dust as such (Stokinger 1953), but smoking in a dusty atmosphere may be regarded as the causative factor. Only Capodaglio *et al.* (1961) reported more long-lasting effects: disturbed pulmonary function after severe exposure in workers who performed a rather heavy work load. The possible use of the reaction of Fuyiwara for discovery of metabolites in urine was discussed by Hassmann (1961).

Dermatological problems hardly arise. If 10% chromic acid is used as a dispersion agent, it should be borne in mind that this substance has primary skin irritating as well as contact-sensitizing properties.

SPECIFIC PREVENTION

The following preventive measures appear to be efficacious:

– Absolute prohibition of smoking in departments, where fluorine-containing polymers are produced or processed; the taking of tobacco into these premises must also be banned.

References p. 180

– If the temperature of the polymers exceeds 200° to 250° special provisions must be made: local ventilation, increasingly powerful as the temperature rises.
– Open fire in the department should be avoided.
– Appliances consisting wholly or partly of fluorine-containing polymers should be marked as such; processing, destroying or burning (in consumer goods industries) of these should also be carried out under special precautions.
– Quantities larger than 50 kg should be stored in special compartments; in case of fire, attention should be paid to protection of the air passages and eyes.
– Refuse should be dealt with separately; it should be burned in furnaces with high chimneys.
– The workmen should receive special instructions regarding hygienic requirements.
– The MAC of polymer dust is 15 mg/m^3 (*Hyg. Guide* 1959). The MAC of HF is 3 p.p.m. = 2 mg/m^3 according to A.C.G.I.H. (1962), and 0.6 p.p.m. = 0.4 mg/m^3 according to Russian authorities (Elkins 1961). The concentration of decomposition products of Teflon should approach zero as far as possible (Johnstone *et al.* 1960). Prescriptions for spray application of Teflon finishes were given by Dupont de Nemours (1962).

REFERENCES

American Conference Governmental Industrial Hygienists, *Threshold Limit Values*, Detroit, Michigan, 1962.

ATKINSON, B. and A. B. TRENWITH, Thermal decomposition of tetrafluoro-ethylene. *J. Chem. Soc.*, (1953) 2082. Ref.: TRUFFERT, 1959.

CAPODAGLIO, E., G. MONARCA and G. DI VITO, Respiratory syndrome from intermediate volatile products of polytetrafluoroethylene. *Rass. Med. Ind.*, 30 (1961) 124. Ref.: *Bull. Hyg.*, 37 (1962) 257.

CAVAGNA, G., M. FINULLI and E. C. VIGLIANI, Experimental study on the pathogenesis of Teflon-fume fever. *Med. Lavoro*, 52 (1961) 251. Ref.: *Bull. Hyg.*, 37 (1962) 144.

CHALLEN, P. J. R., R. J. SHERWOOD and J. BEDFORD, 'Fluon' (polytetrafluoroethylene): a preliminary note on some clinical and environmental observations. *Brit. J. Ind. Med.*, 12 (1955) 177.

CLAYTON, J. W., M. A. DELAPLANE and D. B. HOOD, Toxicity studies with octafluorocyclobutane. *Am. Ind. Hyg. Assoc. J.*, 21 (1960) 382.

DANISHEVSKI, S. L. and M. M. KOGANOV, The toxicology of some fluoro-organic compounds. *Gigiena Truda i Prof. Zabolevaniya*, 5/3 (1961) 3. Ref.: *Bull. Hyg.*, 36 (1961) 1244.

DEHEZ, A., Les composés fluorés organiques et leurs applications en électrotechnique. *Ind. Chem. Belge*, 22 (1957) 263.

Dupont de Nemours, *E. I. Notes on Teflon.* X-592 (undated).

Dupont de Nemours, More about Teflon coatings. *Ind. Finishing*, May 1962, p. 92.

ELKINS, H. B., Maximum acceptable concentrations. *Arch. Environ. Health*, 2 (1961) 45.

French Army and Airforce Authority, L'action toxique de Téflon. *Transform. Plastiques*, 12 (1958) 122.

FRODSHAM, J., Unpublished investigation. I.C.I. Ref.: HARRIS, 1951.

GANCBERG, A., Étude de toxicité d'un revêtement mixte silicones-polytétrafluoroéthylène. *Ind. Chem. Belge*, 24 (1959) 1486.

HAGEMEYER, D. R. and W. STUBBELINE, Physiological activity of fluorocarbon polymers. *Modern Plastics*, 31 (1954) 136. Ref.: TRUFFERT, 1959.

HARRIS, D. K., Polymer-fume fever. *Lancet*, 261 *ii* (1951) 1008.

HARRIS, D. K., Some hazards in the manufacture and use of plastics. *Brit. J. Ind. Med.*, 16 (1959) 221.

HASSMANN, P., Occupational hazards in processing polytetrafluoroethylene (Teflon, Fluon) and polytrifluorchloroethylene (Teflex). *Pracovni Lekar*, 13 (1961) 461. Ref.: *CIS Docum. Dubr:* mz. 172-1962.

Hygienic Guide, Teflon T.F.E.-fluorocarbon resins and their decomposition products. *Am. Ind. Hyg. Assoc J.*, 20 (1959) 436.

Imperial Chemical Industries, Fluon-polytetrafluorcethylene primer and finishes. *I.S.-Note* No. 586, 1959a.

Imperial Chemical Industries, *'Fluon' P.T.F.E.*, 1959b.

JOHNSTONE, R. T. and S. E. MILLER, *Occupational Diseases and Industrial Medicine*, Saunders, Philadelphia, 1960.

LESTER, D. and L. A. GREENBERG, Acute and chronic toxicity of some halogenated derivatives of methane and ethane. *Arch. Ind. Hyg.*, 2 (1950) 335.

MADORSKY, S. L., V. E. HART and V. A. SEDLAK, Thermal decomposition of polymers of tetrafluoroethylene and hydrofluoroethylene *in vitro*. *J. Res. Natl. Bur. Std.*, 51 (1953) 327. Ref.: TRUFFERT, 1959.

National Advisory Council for Aeronautics, Toxicological aspects of the plastic industry. *Memorandum*, Sept. 1956. Ref.: TRUFFERT, 1959.

PATTISON, F. L. M., *Toxic Aliphatic Fluorine Compounds*, Elsevier, Amsterdam, 1959.

PERNIS, B., G. CAVAGNA and M. FINULLI, Degranulation of polymorphonuclear leucocytes exposed to ZnO or Teflon particles. *Med. Lavoro*, 52 (1961) 649. Ref.: *Bull. Hyg.*, 37 (1962) 1130.

SENDROY, J., J. D. O'NEAL and G. C. PITTS, Hazards from thermal decomposition of motor-insulating materials. *Arch. Ind. Hyg.*, 5 (1952) 330.

SHERWOOD, R. J., The hazards of Fluon (polytetrafluoroethylene). *Trans. Assoc. Ind. Med. Officers*, 5 (1955) 10.

SIEGLE, J. and L. MUUS, Pyrolysis of polytetrafluoroethylene. *Lecture Am. Chem. Soc.*, Sept., 1956. Ref.: GANCBERG, 1959.

STOKINGER, H. E., Teflon – a plastic with an inhalation hazard. *Occupational Health*, 13 (1953) 88.

TREON, J. F., F. P. CLEVELAND, E. E. LARSON, J. W. CAPPEL, F. SHAFFER, K. L. STEMMER and R. T. DENHAM, The immediate toxicity of the thermal decomposition products of Teflon and Kel-F. *Rept. Kettering Lab. Univ. Cincinnati*, April, 1954. Ref.: PATTISON, 1959.

TREON, J. F., J. W. CAPPEL, F. P. CLEVELAND, E. E. LARSON, R. W. ATCHLEY and R. T. DENHAM, The toxicity of the products formed by the thermal decomposition of certain organic substances. *Am. Ind. Hyg. Assoc. Quart.*, 16 (1955) 187.

TROYANOWSKI, C., Emploi à chaud du polytétrafluoroéthylène (Teflon), décomposition, toxicité. *Arch. Maladies Prof.*, 20 (1959) 57.

TRUFFERT, L., Aspects toxicologiques de l'industrie des matières plastiques. *Arch. Maladies Prof.*, 20 (1959) 43.

ZAPP, J. A., Toxic and health effects of plastics and resins. *Arch. Environ. Health*, 4 (1962) 335.

ZAPP, J. A., G. LIMPEROS and K. C. BRINKER, Toxicity of pyrolysis products of 'Teflon' tetrafluoroethylene resin. *Lecture Am. Ind. Hyg. Assoc.*, April, 1955. Ref.: HARRIS, 1959.

13

Synthetic fibres

PHYSICO-CHEMICAL PROPERTIES, APPLICATION

The synthetic fibres consist of linear macromolecules; they are produced by synthetic linkage of bifunctional monomolecular compounds. Several groups of synthetic fibres may be distinguished:

Polycondensates

Polyamides
– from adipic acid + hexamethylenediamine (nylon 66, perlon T),
– from ε-caprolactam (nylon 6, perlon L, enkalon),
– from amino undecanic acid (nylon 11).

Polyesters
– from dimethylterephthalate + ethyleneglycol via diglycolester of terephthalic acid (see p. 14) (terylene, dacron, terlenka),
– from dimethylterephthalate + 1,4-dimethylolcyclohexane (kodel).

For technology of some of these polycondensates see Stockburger (1961).

Polymerizates

– from acrylonitrile, as homo- or copolymer (orlon, dralon, acrylon, leacryl), see Chapter 11,

– from vinyl chloride, as homo- or copolymer (rhovyl, vinylon), see Chapter 10,
– from ethylene (nymplex, courlene), see Chapter 10,
– from propene (meraklon, prolene),
– from vinyl alcohol (kuralon, vinylon), see Chapter 10,
– by polyaddition of a di-isocyanate to a di-ol (perlon U, lycra), see Chapter 8.

The spinning process may proceed in two ways:
– from a solution: the polymer is dissolved at increased temperature, mostly in a closed system. The solution is pressed through a spinneret, after which the thread is formed either by a wet (coagulation and washing in several baths) or by a dry procedure (evaporation of the solvent by heated air);
– from a melting phase: the molten polymer is pressed through a spinneret into a heated tunnel. This procedure particularly applies to polyamides and polyesters.

Several auxiliary substances have to be added in one of the stages of production: for instance dyestuffs, solvents, coagulators. Polyacrylonitrile polymers need specific solvents (see p. 165).

The synthetic fibres not only find extensive application as substitutes for natural or semi-natural fibres, but, because of the presence of new properties (for instance chemical resistance), the area of application has been widened considerably.

TOXICOLOGY AND DERMATOLOGY OF POLYAMIDES

From the hygienic viewpoint the compounds ε-caprolactam and hexamethylenediamine deserve special discussion. In addition attention should be paid to a heat-transferring material, a mixture of 26.5% diphenyl and 73.5% diphenyloxide (Dowtherm A, Diphyl, Dinyl), used in the production of polycaprolactam fibres. The polymer products as such (or monomer rests) also may be biologically active, although rarely.

Hexamethylenediamine

In animal experiments (cited by Quooss, 1959) Ceresa *et al.* (1950) observed a slight hemolytic anemia and leucopenia, whereas Martynova (1957) mentioned the occurrence of hypotension, decreased irritability of the nervous system, irritation of mucosae, bronchitis, emphysema, degeneration of myocardium and kidney. The compound has a primary toxic ($pH > 12$) and a sensitizing effect on the skin (Von Oettingen 1958). Gallo *et al.* (1958) examined 20 workers in two factories, exposed to an average of 2 (max. 33) and 6 (max. 132) mg/m^3. In this group 8 subjects suffered from irritation of the mucosae of eyes and upper air passages, whereas one worker had an eczema and an acute liver disease; no blood anomalies were found. The hazard of inhalation of hexamethylenediamine vapour is said to be diminished because of the formation of biologically inactive carbamate in the presence of CO_2. Several cases of occupational contact eczema were described by Duverneuil *et al.* (1952) in workers contacting among other things hexamethylenediamine. Four of them healed after change of job. The authors did not perform patch tests because the substance was considered as a primary caustic. The exposure was not clearly described, and possible different origins of eczema were not excluded. Jansson (1959) investigated two nylon-sensitive women. He obtained negative reactions in patch-testing with 2% hexamethylenediamine in water and with pure adipic acid, but positive results with the low-molecular polyamide made from these basic substances.

ε-Caprolactam = 2-oxohexamethyleneimine

The linear polycaprolactam is formed by heating the compound at 260°. The end-product may contain up to about 10% of the monomer, no by-product being formed.

From the LD_{50}-oral for mice (1.2 g/kg) Hohensee (1951) estimated a lethal oral dose of 70 g for human beings. The com-

References p. 191

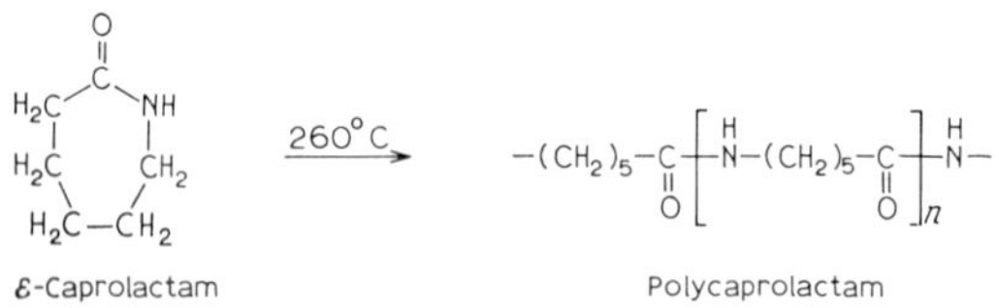

pound proved to be non-toxic for skin and eyes. Chronic oral intake of 150 mg/kg was tolerated by mice. This author concluded that an acute industrial intoxication seemed to be impossible because of the low volatility and the low degree of toxicity. Goldblatt *et al.* (1954) performed extensive animal experiments. Rats tolerated intraperitoneal injections of less than 350 mg/kg; doses of 500–600 mg/kg caused reversible excitation, tremor, decrease of body temperature, whereas 900 mg/kg caused lethal convulsions and disturbed temperature regulation. Intravenous injection of 100–300 mg/kg in rabbits produced a reversible effect similar to picrotoxin. The compound proved to be an antagonist of veronal. Long-lasting oral uptake of 667 mg/kg was tolerated well by rats; an only somewhat diminished growth occurred. Exposure of guinea pigs to 118–261 mg/m^3, 7 h/day for 7 days, caused moderate irritation of the respiratory tract. The human skin tolerated 5% ε-caprolactam in water, alcohol or olive oil, even after repeated application. Goldblatt *et al.* concluded there was a relatively low toxicity, although a potential risk seemed to be present when inhaling high concentrations of ε-caprolactam vapour or dust. Bornmann *et al.* (1959) came to similar conclusions as the previous authors; the LD_{50}-oral for rats was established as 1155 mg/kg.

Hohensee (1951) examined workers from a spinning department (exposure to 61 mg/m^3) and a laboratory (16–17 mg/cm^3). Workers from the first department sometimes mentioned nervous irritability, apprehension, particularly at the end of the working day and after dusty work. The authors also observed epistaxis, inflammation of the upper respiratory tract, dry nose, painful lips, pyrosis, flatulence, heavy feeling in the upper abdomen and a bitter taste. The symptoms rapidly disappeared after a stay in fresh air. Elizarov (1959) examined a group of 67 workers, exposed to less than 17.5 mg/m^3. In addition to general complaints about headache, sleeplessness, decreased appetite, he noted skin diseases which might appear after an exposure of 3 to 4 days: dry glossy skin, loss of the normal sensory perception of the finger tips and thickening of the stratum corneum, with formation of clefts, nail alterations and desquamation. The dermatitis sometimes spread acutely over the whole body, particularly when working in a humid and warm environment. The author did not give any data of patch-testing; the specific agent therefore has not been determined. Schulz *et al.* (1956) considered ε-caprolactam as non-toxic and non-sensitizing for the skin. Elizarov (1959), however, remarked that this substance was strongly hygroscopic, very soluble in fats and weakly toxic. Experiments in rats and rabbits lead to dermatoses with disturbance of keratinization.

From the experimental and occupational data it may be concluded, that, although ε-caprolactam may not be regarded as innocuous, the toxicity and the hazard seem to be rather slight. Although high quantities are being processed, relatively few hygienic consequences seem to have occurred. In the perlon-processing industry Fuchs *et al.* (1957) observed a dermatosis in several workers consisting of deep rhagades in yellow crusty patches situated preferably on volar aspects of thumb and index finger and on the palms. They did not find positive patch tests to a number of substances from the workers' environment and related this dermatosis to the steel-like hardness and the tear-resistance of the finished fibre (to which in the molten state titanium oxide had been added) which, as it were, 'cuts the skin in pieces', if broken fibres have to be torn from the machines or to be knotted. In a factory producing ε-caprolactam by hydration of benzene Antonova *et al.* (1962) examined 79 workers (mostly female). They were exposed to 90–250 mg cyclohexane/m^3 and 1–5 mg nitrocyclohexane/m^3. The authors observed many neurovegetative disorders and an enlargement of the thyroid.

The polyamide polycondensate

Massman *et al.* (1956) examined the biological activity of nylon 66 and perlon L; 5 g of powder was applied intraperitoneally in rabbits. The introduction of perlon caused corpus alienum granulomata, whereas after nylon application a colliquation necrosis was seen, both of them surrounded by an indurated area. No clear evidence of transport to other organs was established.

Gipstein (1941), Prassas (1955), Morris (1960) and Jansson (1959) reported on the relatively very sporadic occurrence of eczemas due to contact with the cured-out nylon or perlon, especially in stockings. This need not be considered strange in the case of perlon because this may contain some unreacted monomer: 0.2–0.3% caprolactam according to Jansson (1959) and 1.5% according to Schulz (1956). Schwann (1963) reported two cases of caprolactam contact eczema due to contact with steelon containing up to 10% free monomer. These patients showed negative patch tests to the cured steelon. In two patients with nylon hypersensitivity, Jansson found negative patch tests with the constituting basic materials adipic acid and hexamethylenediamine, but positive patch tests with the low-molecular reaction product of both these basic substances, which may be present up to about 1% in the cured nylon, according to Stockburger (1961). Müller (1954) reported to have seen urticaria due to the wearing of perlon step-ins.

Diphenyl and diphenyloxide

Deichmann *et al.* (1947) investigated the toxicity of diphenyl. The lethal oral dose (25% in olive oil) for rabbits was 2.41 g/kg and for rats 3.28 g/kg; degeneration of liver, kidney and myocardium occurred, whereas some animals developed slight paralysis of the hind legs and asphyctic convulsions. The vapour pressure was too low to determine the acute inhalatory toxicity. Repeated oral uptake of 1 g diphenyl (in olive oil) did not cause any blood abnormalities, but a total uptake of 4–21 times the acute lethal dose proved to be fatal. Exposure of rats to 40 or 300 mg/m^3 diphenyl (50% on celite), 7 h/day 5 days per week for a period of 64 days, caused serious irritation of the respiratory tract and a slight toxic degeneration of liver and kidney; some animals died. Rabbits tolerated this exposure without undue effects, but mice suffered from distressed respiration at an exposure of only 5 mg/m^3. Deichmann *et al.* recommended from these experimental data a MAC for diphenyl of 0.75 p.p.m. (= 5 mg/m^3). Application of 0.5 g/kg (25% in olive oil) to rabbits' skin, 2 h/day for 5 days, did not cause any local irritation, but systemic toxicity occurred. Diphenyl therefore is able to penetrate the intact skin. Daily oral uptake of 50 or 100 mg for 2 months caused a moderately severe degeneration of liver and kidney in rats; some animals developed papillomata and one of them even a carcinoma of the stomach (Pecchiai *et al.* 1957). Dowtherm A (mixture of 26.5% diphenyl and 73.5% diphenyl oxide) was tolerated by rats in an oral dose of 2 g/kg, but 6 g/kg was lethal; repeated oral uptake of 0.5 g/kg, 5 days per week for 4 weeks, did not cause undue effects, whereas 1 g/kg caused loss of weight. Repeated exposure to 7–10 p.p.m. Dowtherm A vapour, 7 h/day 5 days per week for 6 months, did not give rise to any pathology in three species of animals (Dow 1950). Solomin (1961) determined as odour threshold limit for dinyl (similar to Dowtherm A) a concentration of 0.06 mg/m^3. An exposure to 0.03 mg/m^3 already caused disturbed higher nervous activity in rats. Continuous exposure to 0.2 mg/m^3, 24 h/day for 70 days, resulted in a change in motor chronaxy, porphyrin metabolism, cholinesterase level and blood picture in rats, whereas continuous exposure to 0.01 mg/m^3 did not cause any effects. Because of these results Solomin proposed a maximum allowable concentration (for 24 h) of 0.01 mg dinyl/m^3. Gerarde (1960) observed an increase in

References p. 191

excretion of ethereal sulfates in rats after subcutaneous injection of diphenyl; the significance of this has not yet been evaluated in periodical screening in industry.

Although the animal experiments mentioned above showed a slight to moderate toxicity of diphenyl alone or of its mixture with diphenyloxide, experience from industry has not resulted in any evident disturbances of health in exposed workers. Only one report mentioned some discomfort (Parmeggiani *et al.* 1955). Exposure to 0.1–0.9 p.p.m. resulted in conjunctivitis and pharyngitis; exposure to 1 p.p.m. caused notable irritation of the mucosae, whereas exposure to 3–4 p.p.m. proved to be very disagreeable. The low vapour pressure and the sensory warning signal at low concentration level both decrease the industrial hazard considerably. Skin contact with hot Dowtherm may lead to serious burns, but contact with the liquid at moderate temperatures only results in a temporary slight skin irritation. Goldblatt (1955) proposed a MAC of 0.3 p.p.m. = 2 mg/m^3 for Dowtherm A, which corresponds to 0.5 mg diphenyl and 1.5 mg diphenyl oxide per m^3.

TOXICOLOGY AND DERMATOLOGY OF SATURATED LINEAR POLYESTERS

The synthetic linear polyesters, used as fibre materials, are built up from dimethylterephthalate and a diol. During the first step diglycolester of terephthalic acid is formed (with as a by-product methanol) and a small quantity of oligomers (low-molecular polycondensation products). During the second step polycondensation of the diglycolester takes place (with ethylene glycol as a by-product). Although methanol possesses its well-known toxic hazard, no hygienic consequences have been reported from the synthetic fibre industry. Because of its slight toxicity and of the very low volatility, exposure to dimethylterephthalate hardly bears any hazard. Moreover this compound does not irritate the skin (Lefaux 1952). Ethylene glycol, used as diol, possesses a specific toxic effect on the kidneys by means of the metabolic intermediate oxalic acid. The industrial hazard however is small, because of the low volatility. In sporadic cases chronic exposure has caused irritation of the mucosae, whereas slight non-specific general symptoms were mentioned; some urines contained albumen and erythrocytes (Browning 1953). Troisi (1950) noted a reversible disturbance of the central nervous system (attacks of unconsciousness, nystagmus) in workers exposed to relatively high concentrations, when the compound was being heated to 105°. Toxicological data about dimethylolcyclohexane have not been published. The toxicity may probably be estimated to be at least similar to that of cyclohexane (MAC: 400 p.p.m. = 1400 mg/m³).

TOXICOLOGY AND DERMATOLOGY OF THE POLYMERIZATES

The data regarding acrylonitrile (with its specific solvents dimethylformamide and dimethylsulfoxide), vinyl chloride, vinyl alcohol and isocyanates are discussed in the respective chapters. A moderate narcotic effect may be attributed to ethylene and propylene; Patty (1949) proposed the following MAC values: 5000 p.p.m. (= 6325 mg/m³) and 4000 p.p.m. (= 6880 mg/m³) respectively.

REFERENCES

ANTONOVA, L. T., B. A. KURLYANDSKY, M. M. MELNIKOVA and M. I. SMIRNIKOVA, On the health status of workers engaged in the production of caprolactam from benzol. *Gigiena Truda i Prof. Zabolevaniya*, 6/5 (1962) 14.

BORNMANN, G. and A. LOESER, Studien über Kunststoffe aus ε-caprolactam oder Bisphenol. *Arzneimittel-Forsch.*, 9 (1959) 9.

BROWNING, E., *Toxicity of Industrial Solvents*, H.M.S.O., London, 1953.

CERESA, C. and M. DE BLASIIS, Experimental investigations on hexamethylenediamine poisoning. *Med. Lavoro*, 41 (1950) 78. Ref.: QUOOSS, 1959.

DEICHMANN, W. B., K. V. KITZMILLER, M. DIERKER and S. WITTERUP, Observations on the effects of diphenyl, *o*- and *p*-aminodiphenyl, *o*- and *p*-nitrodiphenyl and dihydroxy-octachlorodiphenyl upon experimental animals. *J. Ind. Hyg.*, 29 (1947) 1.

Dow Chemical Company, *Health hazards and precautions for the safe handling and use of Dowtherm A*, 1950.

DUVERNEUIL, G. and G. BUISSON, Dermites par hexaméthylènediamine. *Arch. Maladies Prof.*, 13 (1952) 389.

ELIZAROV, G. P., Zur Klinik, Prophylaxe und Therapie von Caprolaktam Dermatiden. *Gigiena Truda i Prof. Zabolevaniya*, 3 (1959) 20. Ref.: *Zbl. Arbeitsmed.*, 10 (1960) 176.

FUCHS, F. and H. J. SONNECK, Über einen Hautschaden in der Perlonverarbeitenden Industrie. *Dermatol. Wochschr.*, 136 (1957) 797.

GALLO, G. and L. GHIRINGHELLI, Occupational pathology due to hexamethylenediamine. *Med. Lavoro*, 49 (1958) 683. Ref.: *Excerpta Med. Sect. XVII*, 6 (1960) 106.

GERARDE, H. W., *Toxicology and Biochemistry of Aromatic Hydrocarbons*, Elsevier, Amsterdam, 1960.

GIPSTEIN, E., Dermatitis caused by nylon stockings. *Conn. Med. J.*, 5 (1941) 278.

GOLDBLATT, M. W., Research in industrial health in the chemical industry. *Brit. J. Ind. Med.*, 12 (1955) 1.

GOLDBLATT, M. W., M. E. FARQUHARSON, G. BENNETT and B. M. ASKEW, ε-Caprolactam. *Brit. J. Ind. Med.*, 11 (1954) 1.

HOHENSEE, F., Experience with the manufacture of Perlon-L. *Faserforsch. Textiltechn.*, 2 (1951) 299. Ref.: GOLDBLATT *et al.*, 1954.

JANSSON, H., Zur Frage der Sensibilisierungseigenschaft von Perlon und Nylon Grundsubstanz. *Z. Haut-Geschlechtskr.*, 26 (1959) 37.

LEFAUX, R., *Toxicologie des matières plastiques et des composés macromoléculaires*, Masson, Paris, 1952.

MARTYNOVA, A. P., 'Polyamide'. *Gigiena Truda i prof. Zabolevaniya*, 1/4 (1957) 23. Ref.: QUOOSS, 1959.

MASSMANN, W. and K. PILGRIM, Durch Polyamidstäube hervorgerufene Gewebsreaktionen. *Zbl. Arbeitsmed.*, 6 (1956) 88.

MORRIS, G. E., Nylon-dermatitis. *Berufsdermatosen*, 8 (1960) 155.

MÜLLER, E. M., Urticaria externa und urticarielle Dermatitis durch Perlonhüfthalter. *Z. Haut Geschlechtskr.*, 16 (1954) 5.

OETTINGEN, W. F. VON, *Poisoning; a Guide to Clinical Diagnosis and Treatment*, Saunders, Philadelphia, 1958.

PARMEGGIANI, L. and C. SASSI, Risques et pathologie professionnelle dans la fabrication et le travail de quelques matières plastiques. *Med. Lavoro*, 46 (1955) 14. Ref.: *Arch. Maladies Prof.*, 16 (1955) 507.

PATTY, F. A., *Industrial Hygiene and Toxicology*, Vol. II, Interscience, New York, 1949.

PECCHIAI, L. and U. SAFFIOTTI, Study of the toxicity of diphenyl, diphenyloxide and their mixture (Dowtherm). *Med. Lavoro*, 48 (1957) 247. Ref.: GERARDE, 1960.

PRASSAS, M. N., Dermite bulleuse des pieds provoquée par le nylon pur. *Bull. Soc. Franç. Dermatol. Syphiligraphie*, 62 (1955) 508.

QUOOSS, H., *Gesundheitsgefahren in der Kunstoffindustrie*, Barth, Leipzig, 1959.

SCHULZ, K. H. and W. P. HERMANN, Zur Aetiologie der Perlonstrumpf Ekzemen. *Hautarzt*, 7 (1956) 313.

SCHWANN, J., Berufsstigmata und Dermatitiden bei der Herstellung von Fischnetzen. *Berufsdermatosen*, 11 (1963) 8.

SOLOMIN, G. J., Data substantiating maximum permissible concentration of dinyl in atmospheric air. *Gigiena i Sanit.*, 26/5 (1961) 3.

STOCKBURGER, S., *Chemiefaserkunde*, Econ Verlag, Düsseldorf, 1961.

TROISI, F. M., Chronic intoxication by ethylene glycol vapour. *Brit. J. Ind. Med.*, 7 (1950) 65.

14

Glass-fibre materials

PHYSICO-CHEMICAL PROPERTIES, APPLICATION

Two kinds of glass compounds may be used in reinforced plastics: *E-glass* ('electrical purposes'; alkali-free) and *C-glass* ('chemical purposes'; 11–18% alkalies), both containing 50–65% SiO_2. A short survey of the production process of glass-fibre materials may serve to indicate the points of possible biological activity. Molten glass is pressed through 204 fine holes, producing the same number of glass filaments forming together one strand. A textile size (called 'size') is applied to keep the filaments together (this size contains chiefly oil and starch, sometimes PV acetate). The strand is processed sometimes into staple fibres (chopped fibres, processed like wool), but mainly into continuous fibres. The last type is processed into roving materials or into yarns. Roving fibres are not twisted and twined. These fibres may either be used as such, as glass texture (woven bundles or roving) or as glass mats (the fibres are chopped and kept together by means of a 'binder'). The binder applied in mats is generally an unsaturated polyester (diallylphthalate as cross-linking agent); in a minority of cases phenoplasts or aminoplasts are used (yellow-brown mats). Yarns are twisted and twined, desized (the textile size is removed by heating or by wet treatment) and woven into glass textures. In order to provide a good bond between glass and plastic a reinforcement size (called 'finish') is applied both on roving materials and on yarns, containing an organic group linking with the plastic and an inorganic group linking with the glass materials. The most widely used finishes are: Volan (methacrylate–chrome) finishes (for epoxy resins) and Silane finishes (for polyesters, see *e.g.* Malten 1956). In some cases organic amines are applied as finish; a thin coating of epoxy resin may serve to protect against wetting.

From this short survey it may be concluded that the roving materials and especially the roving mats, offer a greater hazard of biological activity (short fibres, presence of size, binder and finish) than glass materials made from yarns (no size, no binder).

During the handling, measuring and cutting of glass-fibre materials and particularly during machining of reinforced plastics 'glass dust' may be dispersed in the atmosphere. These fine filaments of glass (with additives) in the air are called 'the fly'. According to Lieber (1959) the diametre of glass-fibre materials in dusts is generally 1–20μ, the length 5–10μ; because of a high electrostatic charge, high dust concentrations are not likely. Glass-fibre materials are increasingly applied in reinforced plastics (see Chapter 7), giving the desired mechanical properties to boats, car bodies and many other large or small objects.

EXPERIMENTAL TOXICOLOGY AND DERMATOLOGY

Because of the presence of SiO_2 in glass, the experiments mainly deal with the investigation of silicogenic properties. They can only be reviewed shortly. Intratracheal injection of small glass or silicate particles (Schepers *et al.* 1955, 1961; Gross *et al.* 1956, 1960) showed the relative inertness of these materials, particularly the absence of fibroplastic changes; dispersed alveolar dust foci (glass-filled macrophages) may occur. Inhalation experiments in guinea pigs, rats and rabbits exposed to high concentrations for several months were reported by Schepers *et al.* (1955, 1958, 1959) and Gross *et al.* (1960). Schepers not only exposed the animals to pure glass particles but also to 'fibre-glass plastic' (dust arising from sawing, cutting etc., of

References p. 202

cured reinforced plastics). From these experiments the following conclusions could be drawn:
– Even with high exposure for several months, no progressive fibrosis develops, no collagen is formed; regarding silicogenic properties glass-fibre materials may be considered inert.
– Dust foci may occur and in some experiments damage to the epithelial layer of bronchi and bronchioli is reported; guinea pigs are more susceptible than rats and rabbits (species-sensitivity). In high concentrations glass-fibre materials are probably not completely inert in this respect.
– The presence of a filler (*e.g.* $CaSO_4$, $CaCO_3$) may influence the pulmonary reaction to glass dust.
– Pulmonary tuberculosis is not aggravated by inhalation of glass dust.
– Exposure to concentrations of 50 million particles/$ft.^3$ (about 20 mg/m^3) seems to be a reasonably acceptable level from the viewpoint of comfort (Schepers *et al.* 1958, 1959).

Afterwards Schepers (1962), however, performed a long-lasting experiment in monkeys (Macacus mulatta, fibre-glass plastic, 4.60 $mg/ft.^3$, 8 h/day, 5 days/week, 8 months); he did not see any fibrosis, but observed an increased hilary shadowing, slight increase of pulmonary weight, slight emphysema, a marked perivascular reaction with phagocytosis and lymphatic infiltration. The occurrence of such (reversible) reactions seems to be possible in human beings.

Topical application in the skin and into the eyes (Gross *et al.* 1960; Schepers 1961) also showed the inertness of the materials. In an investigation of the local tissue effects (*e.g.* subcut. inj.) Schepers (1961) proved glass fibres, polyesters and fillers to be relatively inert. The resin and fillers even potentiated to a certain extent the effects of glass. Subcutaneous implantation of glass and plastic caused local fibrosis; implantation of glass alone did not. Tumors were not observed in rats, guinea pigs and rabbits during an observation time of 18 months.

As early as 1942, Sulzberger *et al.* thoroughly investigated the effects of fibre glass on animal and human skin. As the results of their investigations in animals largely corresponded to those in human volunteers, only the latter are cited here. The human subjects were rubbed, over periods varying from 7 to 19 days, with two fibre-glass materials in wool-like form, or two fibre-glass textile materials in fabric form, using absorbent cotton as control. These materials were rubbed in on 3 sides on both forearms for 2 minutes every day. In addition to the sensory disturbances at the time of rubbing, there was some pain and discomfort for some time after application, but astonishingly enough even when the objective signs of skin irritation increased with each rubbing, the subjective manifestations were not intensified. The objective reactions consisted of erythema, swelling, pinhead sized papules soon after rubbing, followed within a few hours by erythema, scaling and varying degrees of crusting. Later on, after several rubbings, persisting papules, lichenification, scaling and varying degrees of hyper-pigmentation were observed. No marked degree of sensitization was produced to any of the materials even under the severe conditions of the original exposure. The histologic changes in all sites, including the sites rubbed with absorbent cotton, were of approximately the same type: the epidermis was generally found to be intact, no glass spicules and no foreign-body reaction in the cutis were seen, showing that no fragment had penetrated through the epidermis.

INDUSTRIAL TOXICOLOGY

Experiences with a forerunner of the modern glass fibres, glass wool applied as insulating material, have been reported by Dhers *et al.* (1946), Desoille *et al.* (1946) and Koelsch (1956): silicosis did not occur, but discomfort (and sometimes even lung abscesses, Murphy 1961) was caused by irritation of the mucosae of eyes and air passages. In the plastics industry, nowadays, ventilation is probably more efficient than during insulating

References p. 202

work in former days, but on the other hand the particle size is considerably smaller. Still very few disturbances of health attributed to glass-fibre materials (apart from skin affections) have been reported from the plastics industry. Only Mungo (1960) referred to rhinitis, blepharoconjunctivitis, pharyngitis, increased bronchovascular shadowing; some workers complained of burning irritation of eyes and nose and gastric disorders. It is not very clear whether the reported symptoms should be attributed to glass-fibre exposure only. Russian authors (Tuchenko *et al.* 1961) objected to the acceptable concentration suggested by Schepers; they proposed a value of 3 mg/m^3, which is generally easily exceeded during cutting and application of glass materials and particularly during machining of the cured products.

INDUSTRIAL DERMATOLOGY

Schwartz *et al.* (1943) reported on skin hazards in the manufacture of glass wool and thread. The wool was sprayed with a phenol-formaldehyde binder diluted with a pine-product solvent; after passing the curing and drying ovens this resin was completely cured and thus did no harm. In the manufacture of glass wool, glass slugs (which are small particles of imperfectly formed fibres) are produced. When glass wool is firmly handled the slugs can be felt and can penetrate the skin. The employees working at the loading sections often had fissures, cuts and scaling of the fingers, hands and wrists. Some developed redness and itching due to irritation by the slugs. The majority did not seem to be troubled by handling the wool and preferred not to wear gloves or protective clothing of any kind. A rubber compound (binder in glass wool for air filtration) and tricresyl phosphate (added to glass wool as dust adhesive) gave no complaints. The fibres were coated with a layer of liquid binder (mixture of starch, polyvinyl alcohol and a substituted pyrazine compound). Twelve out of 65 workers suffered from 'dermatitis' which appeared from 2 to 8 weeks after first contact with the binder. Seven of them were patch-tested with the binder, with a positive result in 3. Tolerance was acquired by several workers. The binder was considered to be the sensitizing agent. Desoille *et al.* (1946) observed in glass-fibre insulators that wearing of close fitting clothes increased the pruritus at the wrists and neck. This pruritus began shortly after starting the work and continued for some hours after work stopped if no shower baths were taken and work clothes were not changed. A number of workers seemed to be more susceptible, but as a rule the majority of the workers got used to the itch. In a small number of workers punctate or diffuse redness on the pruritic sites were seen, sometimes with development of micropapules. These efflorescences started some hours after the beginning of the pruritus, and continued sometimes for several days or weeks even after contact with glass-fibre spicules was stopped. Histologically the glass spicules could be demonstrated penetrating into the epithelium, cutis-granulomata not being mentioned. Saipt (1953) seems to be the only author in the literature accessible to us, who mentioned the formation of granulomatous nodules in the cutis. Miescher and Jordi (both cited by Koelsch 1956) reported cases of eczema and corneal ulcers due to glass spicules. McKenna *et al.* (1958) reported on 126 operatives in the manufacture of continuous glass fibre which, for textile use, was treated with dextrin, gelatin, polyvinyl alcohol, borax, hydrogenated vegetable oil, emulsifying agent, cationic agent and formaldehyde, and for the reinforcement of plastic with polyvinyl acetate, dibutylphthalate, cationic agent, softener, Vitrafix (= solution of methacrylatochromic chloride in an isopropyl-acetone–water solvent), and vinyltrichlorosilane. In 8 cases they saw paronychia with secondary malformation of the nails presumably due to glass spicules. In 14 cases they observed folliculitis of the dorsum of the feet, lower third of the legs, forearms and occasionally of the hands, dull red papular or papulopustular in appearance, not itching and with respect to exacerbation and complete remission unrelated to work, probably due to the hydro-

References p. 202

genated vegetable oils and organic chemicals in the emulsions. No contact sensitizations were observed. Erwin (1947) described the manufacture of ducts of fibre-glass fabric and Plaskon resin processed with styrene, benzoyl peroxide, tricresyl phosphate, antimony oxide and chloraffin. He observed a number of workers with contact eczema presumably due to the plastic binder of the fibre glass, as may be concluded from beneficial transfer to another shop (no ingredients, no patch test reported). During a 6-year survey of an aircraft plant Malten did not observe any cases of contact eczema due to fibre glass (finished either with a chrome methacrylate compound (Volan A = Treatment T5) or with a vinyl chlorosilane compound), used as reinforcement of unsaturated polyester resins. However, in a few cases papular dermatitis was observed on the volar aspects of the forearms, starting during the first days or weeks of exposure and generally subsiding a couple of weeks later when the man got 'hardened' against that itchy feeling ('as if they had visited a barber's shop'). Foreign body granulomata were never observed. As soon as it was realized that this dermatitis might prepare the way for a contact sensitization to one of the unsaturated polyester ingredients, working with resins was strictly separated from handling glass-fibre materials. We feel this to be the most important preventive measure against contact sensitization to polyester resin ingredients, which from that very moment have disappeared in the factory observed. White (1954) pointed out the possibility of irritation problems being carried over to subsequent assembly operations because of dust adhering to fabricated parts. Silicon granulomas as described by Crossland (1955) apparently never occur in this type of work.

SPECIFIC PREVENTION

To prevent the 'fly', White (1954) advised vacuum exhaustion with an ordinary household vacuum cleaner with an appropriately designed and placed suction nozzle. An exhaust system will be unnecessary if the equipment and work is such that the operation can be conducted under a stream of water or other coolant. Erwin (1947) reported that by modifying the process so that the pieces are moistened with the binder before cutting, the number of dispersed particles, and the irritation they cause, markedly decreased in comparison with the process when the pieces were cut dry, pasted on, then provided with the solution. The carrying of dust adhering to machined parts is prevented by dip-washing of the parts in a very thin solution of some common liquid wax and a convenient solvent such as naphtha (White 1954).

Erwin (1947) observed that wherever protective (plastic foil) sleeves were available, they seemed to provide no more benefit than long-sleeved clothing, except in the shop where the plaster is removed and the edge burred. The workmen should wear clothing that is loose at the neck, wrists and ankles, and should have washing facilities with a non-abrasive lanolated cleansing wetting agent before meals and at the end of each shift. Sometimes shower baths are considered necessary; the workmen should afterwards change their working clothes. Protective creams have been found to help somewhat. Workers handling glass fibres should not touch sensitizing chemicals.

Hess (1958) advised rubbing the skin with a very dilute sodium carbonate or sodium phosphate solution (1–2%), some time before starting work with glass-fibre materials, in order to harden the stratum corneum and to make it more resistant against introduction of spicules.

In cutting glass-fibre cloth, the table leaf should be furnished with slit-like exhaust devices along the inner sides of the elevated rims.

References p. 202

REFERENCES

CROSSLAND, P. M., Silicon granuloma of the skin. *Arch. Dermatol. Syphilol.*, 71 (1955) 457.

DESOILLE, H. and V. DHERS, Enquête sur les conditions du travail des ouvriers calori-fugeurs employant la fibre de verre. *Arch. Maladies Prof.*, 7 (1946) 332.

DHERS, V., J. PELLERAT, J. COUDERT and L. ROCHE, La pathologie professionnelle de la filature des fibres de verre; l'industrie de la fibre de verre. *Arch. Maladies Prof.*, 7 (1946) 19.

ERWIN, J. R., Fiberglass plastics – industrial medical aspects and experiences. *Ind. Med.*, 16 (1947) 439.

GROSS, P., M. L. WESTRICK, H. H. SCHRENK and J. M. MCCERNEY, The effect of a synthetic ceramic fiber dust upon the lungs of rats. *Arch. Ind. Health*, 13 (1956) 161.

GROSS, P., M. L. WESTRICK and J. M. MCCERNEY, Glass dust: a study of its biologic effects. *Arch. Ind. Health*, 21 (1960) 10.

HESS, W., Glasfaserverstärkte Kunststoffe – neue Werkstoffe für die Metallindustrie. *Technica*, 6 and 7, Birkhäuser Verlag, Basel, 1958.

KOELSCH, F., Untersuchungen über Gesundheitsschädigungen durch Glaswolle und Steinwolle. *Zbl. Arbeitsmed.*, 6 (1956) 181.

LIEBER, E. E., Medical hazards of dust and vapour in the plastic industry. *Reinforced Plastics*, 3 (1959) 18.

MCKENNA, W. B., J. F. F. SMITH and D. A. MCLEAN, Dermatoses in the manufacture of glass fibre. *Brit. J. Ind. Med.*, 15 (1958) 47.

MUNGO, A., Affections of persons working in the manufacture of stratified glass wool products. *Folia Med. (Naples)*, 43 (1960) 962. Ref.: *Excerpta Med. Sect. XVII*, 7 (1961) 712.

MURPHY, G. B., Fiber glass pneumoconiosis. *Arch. Environ. Health*, 3 (1961) 704.

SAIPT, O., Zu den Glaswollschäden der Haut. *Hautarzt*, 4 (1953) 175.

SCHEPERS, G. W. H., The biological action of glass wool; studies on experimental pulmonary histopathology. *Arch. Ind. Health*, 12 (1955) 280.

SCHEPERS, G. W. H., The influence of fiberglass plastic dust on tuberculosis, *Am. Rev. Tuberc. Pulmonary Diseases*, 78 (1958) 512.

SCHEPERS, G. W. H., The pulmonary reaction to sheet fiberglass-plastic dust. *Am. Ind. Hyg. Assoc. J.*, 20 (1959) 73.

SCHEPERS, G. W. H., The pathogenicity of glass-reinforced plastics. *Arch. Environ. Health*, 2 (1961) 620.

SCHEPERS, G. W. H., Reaction of monkey lung to siliceous dust. *Arch. Environ. Health*, 5 (1962) 278.

SCHEPERS, G. W. H. and A. B. DELAHANT, An experimental study of the effects of glass wool on animal lungs. *Arch. Ind. Health*, 12 (1955) 276.

SCHEPERS, G. W. H., T. M. DURKAN, A. B. DELAHANT, A. J. REDLIN, J. G. SCHMIDT, F. T. CREEDON, J. W. JACOBSON and D. A. BAILEY, The biological action of fiberglass-plastic dust. *Arch. Ind. Health*, 18 (1958) 34.

SCHWARTZ, L. and I. BOTVINICK, Skin hazards in manufacture of glass wool and thread. *Ind. Med.*, 12 (1943) 143.

SULZBERGER, M. and R. BAER, The effects of fiberglass on animal and human skin. *Ind. Med.*, 11 (1942) 483.

TUCHENKO, M. M. and P. V. BIDYAKOV, Issues of industrial hygiene in the production of glass plastics. *Gigiena Truda i Prof. Zabolevaniya*, 5/10 (1961) 20.

WHITE, R. B., Dust irritation problems in fabricating reinforced plastics. *Modern Plastics*, 31 (1954) 129.

15

Amorphous silicon dioxide

PHYSICO-CHEMICAL PROPERTIES, APPLICATION

Amorphous silicon dioxide (SiO_2) differs from the well-known crystalline silica not only in its physical structure. The particle size is also generally much smaller: 3–400 mμ (30–4000 Å). The material is therefore voluminous and light and very readily dispersed. The particles easily agglomerate into aggregates, but the percentage (in weight) respirable dust was in an experiment by Byers *et al.* (1961) still 25–40. Studies made with an electronic microscope proved the aggregates to consist of numerous very small particles (Roberts 1955).

Amorphous SiO_2 is prepared in different ways: burning $SiCl_4$ in H_2 and air is the general procedure, but acid precipitation of a solution of sodium silicate is also used. It is not certain whether 'flame silica' has exactly the same properties as 'precipitated silica'.

Amorphous SiO_2 is increasingly becoming applied as a filler in plastics, rubbers and paints.

EXPERIMENTAL TOXICOLOGY AND DERMATOLOGY

Because of the relationship to crystalline silica, in most experiments amorphous silicon dioxide has been studied with a view to silicogenic properties.

Schepers *et al.* (1957) investigated the effects of *inhalation* of flame silica (32–4000 Å), 1.5 mg/ft^3. throughout a period of 12 months in rats. The toxicity was considerable: 74% died between the 4th and the 9th month. The deposition of SiO_2 in the lungs increased with time, but decreased again when the exposure had been stopped. No progressive fibrosis was seen, but focal emphysema and particularly disturbance of pulmonary circulation (obstruction of the vessels by cellular 'cuffs' and intramural occlusion of capillaries by cell agglomerations) occurred. Similar effects were seen in guinea pigs, although mortality was less. In rabbits, a progressive functional disturbance became evident: increase of hemoglobin, number of erythrocytes, hematocrit value and pressure in left and right cardiac ventricle (in one case even cor pulmonale), in addition to (peri)bronchitis, intramural cellular infiltrations, perivascular noduli, ductal stenosis and emphysema. Most of these phenomena were reversible and non-progressive. In exposed rats, guinea pigs and rabbits a strikingly low frequency of non-specific lung infections was seen. Experimental tuberculosis in guinea pigs was also favourably influenced. In a long-lasting ($3\frac{1}{2}$ years) inhalation experiment on rabbits, Gärtner (1952) had already noted similar results. He, however, mentioned also the presence of granulomas (macrophages) and adenoma formation, which resembled phenomena seen in berylliosis and sarcoidosis (Boeck). According to Klosterkötter *et al.* (1952, 1953) the elimination rate is much increased in comparison with crystalline silica, not because of the smaller particle size, but chiefly because of the much greater solubility.

In 1962 Schepers reported an experiment on monkeys (8 h/day, 5 day/week, 12 months, 0.43 mg SiO_2/ft.^{3}, 200 Å). The animals became lethargic, less active; the lungs showed a definite destructive emphysema, because the alveolar septa broke down, with cardiac hypertrophy.

Experiments with *intratracheal injection* of flame silica in rats and guinea pigs were made by several authors (Jötten *et al.* 1952; Klosterkötter 1952; Policard *et al.* 1954; Schepers *et al.*

References p. 209

1957; Schlipköter *et al.* 1956, 1957). The results may be summarized as follows: amorphous SiO_2 is much more soluble than crystalline SiO_2; this explains the greater toxicity and the smaller fibroplastic potency; fibroplasia however may occur if a low level of SiO_2 can be maintained for a certain period. The fibroplastic potency may be enhanced by ribonucleinic acid (Schlipköter *et al.* 1956).

Similar conclusions could be drawn from *intraperitoneal* injections (Jötten *et al.* 1952; Lundgren *et al.* 1953; Rüttner *et al.* 1954; Policard *et al.* 1954; Schlipköter *et al.* 1956; Schepers *et al.* 1957; Charbonnier 1958): fibroplasia occurred if either amorphous SiO_2 was eliminated relatively slowly (large particle size) or a low level could be maintained for a certain period by repeated injections or by special techniques (air-pouch technique, Löblich *et al.* 1961).

Intravenous injection (Klosterkötter 1953a; King 1954; Swensson *et al.* 1956; Schepers *et al.* 1957) confirmed the greater toxicity of amorphous silica in contrast to the crystalline analogue. The toxicity increased with decreasing particle size.

Oral intake of 50 mg flame silica by rats for a period of 3 months did not produce any toxic effects.

Skin irritation did not appear after local application. Injection into the conjunctiva and corpus vitreum was very corrosive (Gärtner *et al.* 1953); subcutaneous injection (Koch 1949) did not produce fibroplasia, but cysts. By combination with compounds which retarded the elimination (polyvinylpyrrolidone, diamond dust, coating with trimethylchlorosilane), fibroplasia could be established (Klosterkötter 1953b; Schiller, 1955; Strecker, 1956, 1961). Strecker (1961) mentioned the occurrence of pathologic alterations in the distal tubuli of the kidney as a result of precipitation of polysilicic acid in animals exposed to Aerosil.

In the above-mentioned investigations flame silica was used. Byers *et al.* (1961) did some experiments with precipitated silica. The acute toxicity (i.v. injection in rats) proved to be less for precipitated SiO_2; the results of intratracheal injection generally corresponded with the data mentioned above.

From the experimental data, the following *conclusions* may be drawn regarding amorphous SiO_2.

It does not produce the progressive fibrosis typical of crystalline silica. Fibroplastic potency is present if the elimination is retarded and a long-lasting level of SiO_2 is maintained. Toxicity increases with the solubility and is far greater than the toxicity of crystalline SiO_2. Oxygen uptake may be interfered with as a result of a disturbance of the circulation. Destructive emphysema and pulmonary hypertension with secondary cardiac failure occurred.

The animals were exposed to high concentrations. Moreover, a species sensitivity was present. It is not clear whether the above-mentioned conclusions are also valid with regard to human beings.

INDUSTRIAL TOXICOLOGY AND DERMATOLOGY

Although amorphous SiO_2 has been increasingly used in industry, comparatively few signs and symptoms have been reported. Schepers *et al.* (1957) mentioned the occurrence of some signs of bronchitis; moreover they indicated the possibility of altering the reaction of pulmonary tissue to beryllium. Amorphous SiO_2 has also been suspected as the cause of Shavers' disease (heating of bauxite with a content of 7% silica yields a smoke with 32% amorphous SiO_2, Jephcott 1950).

Volk (1960) made a follow-up of 215 workers in a flame silica (50–400 Å) producing factory over a period of 12 years; 44 workers were employed for over 10 years. The dust concentrations were in some departments 2–7 mg/m^3. She did not find any case of silicosis. In two workers, an interlobar pleuritis has been observed but a causal relationship with exposure could not be definitely established. The observation period is still too short to exclude the possibility of silicosis after many years of exposure.

References p. 209

Plumkett *et al.* (1962) investigated 78 workers, exposed for an average of 4.75 years (1–16.5 years) to Hi-Sil (precipitated amorphous SiO_2, 22–30 mμ) and Silene (calcium silicate pigment, 30 mμ). The combined exposure concentration was on average 0.21 mg/ft.^{3} ($<$ 0.01–1.65 mg/ft.^{3}) in the general atmosphere of the factory, and 1.01 mg/ft.^{3} ($<$ 0.01–5.77 mg/ft.^{3}) for the bag-parkers. No effect on health and no silicosis was observed.

If amorphous or crystalline silicon happens to enter traumatic skin wounds, silicon granuloma formation of the skin may ensue after an average latency period of 15 years, according to Crossland (1955). No correlation can be made between the degree of pathogenicity of a particular silicon compound and the severity of reaction or length of latency. Clinically nodular lesions (often in scars) can be observed (compatible with those of other foreign body granulomas and resembling keloids, nodular syphilides or various skin tumors) or small purplish lichen ruber-like papules may occur. Microscopically all lesions show tubercle formation without caseation. The only means of identifying anisotropic crystalline material (lying free in the tissue or within giant cells or both) as being silicon is a microdissection technique combined with roentgen absorption spectrography (Engström technique cited by Crossland 1955).

With regard to the experience from industry and the above-mentioned experimental data (no silicosis after very long exposure), it may be concluded that the risk of silicosis is zero to minimal. Amorphous silicon dioxide however is not inert. A possibility of damage to lung tissues and functional disturbance of oxygen uptake probably exists.

SPECIFIC PREVENTION

It is advisable to regard the compound as an undesirable aspecific dust, and to prevent inhalation as far as reasonably possible. Workers with chronic respiratory diseases should not be exposed. Employees should be examined periodically.

REFERENCES

BYERS, P. D. and J. C. GAGE, The toxicity of precipitated silica. *Brit. J. Ind. Med.*, 18 (1961) 295.

CHARBONNIER, J., Toxicité et nocivité de silices amorphes en relation avec leur finesse et leur vitesse de dissolution. In K. W. JÖTTEN und W. KLOSTERKÖTTER (Eds.), *Die Staublungerkrankungen*, Bd. 3, Steinkopff, Darmstadt, Wissenschaftliche Forschungsberichte, Bd. 66, 1958, p. 215.

CROSSLAND, P. M., Silicon granuloma of the skin. *Arch. Dermatol. Syphilol.*, 71 (1955) 457.

GÄRTNER, H., Untersuchungen über die Wirkung feinkörniger, amorpher Kieselsäure in der Lunge von Kaninchen. *Arch. Hyg. Bakteriol.*, 136 (1952) 451.

GÄRTNER, H. and H. KRÜMMELL, Untersuchungen über die Wirkung der Kieselsäure am Kaninchenauge. *Arch. Hyg. Bakteriol.*, 137 (1953) 292.

JEPHCOTT, C. M., Chemical aspects of Shaver's disease. In *Pneumoconiosis*, Ed. J. VERWALD, Hoeber, New York, 1950.

JÖTTEN, K. W. and W. KLOSTERKÖTTER, Die Bedeutung der Löslichkeit der Kieselsäure auf das Zustandekommen der Pneumokoniosen. *Arch. Hyg. Bakteriol.*, 136 (1952) 1.

KING, E. J., La silicose. *Prévention Accid. Contr. Techn.*, 8 (1954) 105.

KLOSTERKÖTTER, W., Tierexperimenteller Beitrag zur Frage der toxischen Wirkung molekulargelöster Kieselsäure. *Arch. Hyg. Bakteriol.*, 136 (1952) 188.

KLOSTERKÖTTER, W., Über Gefässwirkung kolloidaler und molekular gelöster Kieselsäure. *Arch. Hyg. Bakteriol.*, 137 (1953) 69.

KLOSTERKÖTTER, W. and K. W. JÖTTEN, Die Wirkung verschiedener Kieselsäure Formen im Tierexperiment. *Arch. Hyg. Bakteriol.*, 137 (1953) 625.

KOCH, W., Die Wirkung verschiedener Kieselsäureformen im sensibilisierten Tierorganismus. *Frankfurter Z. Pathol.*, 60 (1949) 58. Ref.: RÜTTNER *et al.*, 1954.

LÖBLICH, H. J. and K. WERKLE, Vergleichende qualitative und quantitative Untersuchungen über die Entwicklung des Quarz- und Aerosilgranuloms. *Beitr. Silikose-Forsch.*, 73 (1961) 37. Ref.: *Bull. Hyg.*, 37 (1962) 709.

LUNDGREN, K. D. and A. SWENSSON, Experimental investigations on the significance of the size of the particles in the reactions of the peritoneum to amorphous silica. *Acta Med. Scand.*, 145 (1953) 84.

PLUMKETT, E. R. and B. J. DE WITT, Occupational exposure to Hi-Sil and Silene. *Arch. Environ. Health.*, 5 (1962) 469.

POLICARD, A. and A. COLLET, Toxic and fibrosing action of submicroscopic particles of amorphous silica. *Arch. Ind. Hyg.*, 9 (1954) 389.

ROBERTS, M. L., Relationship of particle count, weight, shape and size of air-borne dusts. *Arch. Ind. Health*, 12 (1955) 361.

RÜTTNER, J. R., W. WILLY and A. BAUMANN, Tierexperimentelle Studien zur Wirkung von amorpher kolloidaler und kristalliner Kieselsäure. *Schweiz. Z. Pathol.*, 17 (1954) 352.

SCHEPERS, G. W. H., Reaction of monkey lung to siliceous dust. *Arch. Environ. Health.*, 5 (1962) 278.

SCHEPERS, G. W. H., T. M. DURKAN, A. B. DELAHANT, F. T. CREEDON and A. J. REDLIN, The biological action of Degussa submicron amorphous silica dust (Dow corning silica). *Arch. Ind. Health*, 16 (1957) 125, 203, 280, 363 and 499.

SCHILLER, E., Zur Pathogenese der Silikose; Löslichkeit plus Fremdkörper Wirkung. *Arch. Gewerbepathol. Gewerbehyg.*, 14 (1955) 1.

SCHLIPKÖTER, H. W. and I. ROTHES, Die Entstehung einer nodulären Fibrose nach intratrachealer Injektion eines Kieselsäuresols in Rattenlungen. *Z. Hyg. Infektionskrankh.*, 142 (1956) 487.

SCHLIPKÖTER, H. W., I. ROTHES and A. J. DEFESCHE, Einfluss des Dispersionsgrades einer feinkörnigen amorphen Kieselsäure auf die biologische Wirkung bei intratrachealen Rattenversuchen. *Z. Hyg. Infektionskrankh.*, 143 (1957) 533.

STRECKER, F. J., Verhalten von Trimethylsilyl-aerosil im Tierversuch. *Beiträge zur Silikose-Forschung*, *Grundfragen* II, Bergbau Berufsgenossenschaft, Bochum, 1956, p. 343.

STRECKER, F. J., Discussion and remark, in *Beiträge zur Silikose-Forschung*, *Grundfragen* IV, Bergbau Berufsgenossenschaft, Bochum, 1961, p. 150.

SWENSSON, A., J. GLOMME and G. BLOOM, On the toxicity of silica particles. *Arch. Ind. Health*, 14 (1956) 482.

VOLK, H., The health of workers in a plant making dispersed silica. *Arch. Environ. Health*, 1 (1960) 125.

16

Organic peroxides

PHYSICO-CHEMICAL PROPERTIES, APPLICATION

Organic peroxides are compounds related to hydrogen peroxide (HOOH); one (hydroperoxide = ROOH) or both (ROOR) H-atoms are substituted by organic groups. They are nonvolatile, very reactive oxidizing agents, readily forming organic radicals. This property is made use of in polymerization reactions (see Chapter 1). The organic peroxides are not 'genuine' catalysers; they take part in the chemical reaction, and are, therefore, not present as such in the high-polymer end-products. The disintegration into radicals may be promoted by temperature, but also by accelerators (*e.g.* Co-naphthenate), as used in the cold-curing of unsaturated polyesters. Reducing agents (stabilizers, inhibitors) may be added to prevent or retard the production of radicals. Organic peroxides are applied as catalysers for polymerization reaction; they are dispersed in plastifiers (*e.g.* dimethyl phthalate) or organic solvents. Mixtures of peroxides and accelerators are very explosive; the handling instructions of the delivering firms should be carefully observed.

EXPERIMENTAL TOXICOLOGY AND DERMATOLOGY

As the hazard to the *eyes* proved to be the main hygienic problem, most work has been concentrated on this issue. Küchle (1958) applied several peroxides as solution, paste or powder

References p. 216

in the eyes of rabbits; in the experiments with paste or powder he washed out the eyes with water 1 min after application. The eyes were observed for six weeks. The resulting effects may be classified as follows:

– *minor reactions (L):* temporary vascular injection, slight chemosis healing within 2 days;

– *moderate reactions (M):* chemosis and purulent conjunctivitis, healing within 3 weeks without residual effects;

– *severe reactions (S):* residual turbidity of cornea, staphyloma, perforation, symblepharon or total destruction.

The results as to different peroxides have been compiled in Table 6. The biological activity parallels the chemical activity; aged mixtures of cyclohexanone peroxide are therefore more aggressive than recently prepared ones (presumably so because of a higher percentage of hydroperoxides). Küchle also investigated some first aid measures. Intensive washing out with tap water was of some use 30 sec after application, but washing after 60 sec was of no avail. In some cases a solution of 2% sodium bicarbonate proved to be superior to tap water; the same effect was sometimes seen from 10% vitamin C (reducing compound) and 0.5% zincum sulfuricum. A 10% solution of tannine was of hardly any use and a 2% vitamin A-containing oil definitely promoted the deleterious effects of the peroxides. Floyd *et al.* (1958) arrived at similar results. The effects of peroxides in 5, 10, 15 and 20% solutions (as used in some paints) have been investigated by Van Rees *et al.* (1958). The solvent acetone as such produced a slight reversible irritation in contrast to ethyl acetate, and low concentrations of peroxides in the latter solvent were less irritating than similar concentrations in acetone.

The *systemic toxicity* has been investigated by Horgan *et al.* (1957) and by Floyd *et al.* (1958). Methyl ethyl ketone peroxide (probably a mixture of ROOH and ROOR) was the most toxic compound; *tert.*-butyl hydroperoxide and cumene hydroperoxide proved to be moderately toxic, whereas di-*tert.*-butyl peroxide was relatively harmless to slightly toxic. For some peroxides

TABLE 6

THE EFFECT OF ORGANIC PEROXIDES ON RABBITS' EYES, COMPILED FROM THE EXPERIMENTAL DATA OF KÜCHLE AND OF FLOYD *et al.*

Peroxide	*Vehicle and concentration*	*Effect* *L.*	*M.*	*S.*
Lauroyl peroxide	as powder	+	–	–
Benzoyl peroxide	as powder 93%	+	–	–
	as paste 50%	+	–	–
Di-*tert*.-butyl peroxide	liquid	+	–	–
tert.-Butyl hydroperoxide	75% solution	–	–	+
	35% in propylene glycol	–	–	+
	7% in propylene glycol	+	–	–
tert.-Butyl perbenzoate	50% in dimethyl phthalate	+	–	–
tert.-Butyl peracetate	50% in dimethyl phthalate	–	+	–
Cyclohexanone peroxide	50% in cyclohexanone	–	–	+
	50% in dimethyl phthalate	–	–	+
	40% liquid	–	–	+
Dicumyl peroxide	?	–	+	–
Cumene hydroperoxide	70% liquid	–	–	+
	10% in propylene glycol	–	–	+
	1% in propylene glycol	+	–	–
Diacetyl peroxide	30% in dimethyl phthalate	–	–	+
Methylethyl ketone peroxide	4% in dimethyl phthalate	–	–	+
	3% in dimethyl phthalate	–	–	+
	0.6% in dimethyl phthalate	+	–	–

References p. 216

repeated sublethal doses either orally or intraperitoneally resulted in cumulative effects ending in the death of some animals. The compounds which were irritating to the eyes affected the skin in a similar way.

INDUSTRIAL TOXICOLOGY

No systemic effects have been reported, probably owing to the low volatility. Moreover the compounds are usually applied in relatively small amounts. Splashes in the eyes, however, do occur, although serious consequences have not yet been reported in the literature. The warning and first-aid instructions of the delivering firms probably saved quite a few eyes. Kayanovitch *et al.* (1962) reported neurovegetative symptoms, irritations of the respiratory tract and disturbances of ventilation function in addition to monocytosis in workers exposed to phosgene (below 4–5 mg/m^3) and chlorobenzoyl (below 1 mg/m^3) in the production of benzoyl peroxide.

INDUSTRIAL DERMATOLOGY

Literature references are very scarce. Benzoyl peroxide has been cited (Grosfeld 1951) as a rather frequent sensitizer in bakers during the period it was used to improve flour. Malten (1956) observed 3 cases of contact eczema due to the use of 50% benzoyl peroxide in a phthalate plasticizer out of a group of 30 workers (who handled unsaturated polyester resins during the stage of experimental production of aircraft devices), one of them also being sensitized to methyl ethyl ketone hydroperoxide (50% in dimethyl phthalate). During the same period two others of the same group appeared to be sensitized to cyclohexanone hydroperoxide (60% in tricresyl phosphate, *cf.* Table 1, p. 79). There were no reactions to the cited plasticizers. These workers were changed over to work with different types of resins occurring in the same factory hall and healed uneventfully.

During that phase of production these organic peroxide mixtures were used in unsaturated polyester–glass fibre constructions applied with bare hand. After introduction of sound hygienic measures and the use of flexible plastic applicators to avoid handling, no more cases were seen during a 5-year observation period in which more people worked with ever increasing quantities of these substances. The approximate toxic concentrations in 24-h patch tests and the testing concentrations to discover sensitizations for the industrial mixtures which were used in 1955, were as follows:

	Toxic conc.	*Testing conc.*
50% benzoyl peroxide in a phthalate dissolved in acetone	10%	5%
50% methyl ethyl ketone hydroperoxide in dimethyl phthalate, dissolved in acetone	1%	½%
60% cyclohexanone hydroperoxide in tricresyl phosphate, dissolved in alcohol	1%	½%

Key (1961) mentioned primary skin irritation from methyl ethyl ketone peroxide (also sensitizer), cumene hydroperoxide, benzoyl peroxide (also sensitizer), lauryl peroxide, 2,4-dichlorobenzoyl peroxide, *p*-chlorobenzoyl peroxide, di-*tert*.-butyldiperphthalate, *tert*.-butyl perbenzoate, *tert*.-butyl hydroperoxide (cyclohexanone peroxide is only named a sensitizer). Compared with the toxic eye effects summarized in Table 6, a striking incongruity exists concerning benzoyl peroxide and *tert*.-butyl perbenzoate: skin irritants which have a low irritant effect upon rabbit eyes. The cause of this incongruity may be a difference in composition of the industrial compounds under investigation.

References p. 216

SPECIFIC PREVENTION

The following should be adhered to (see also *Chem. Safety Data Sheet* SD-81, 1960):

– Use of goggles, face-masks etc., when pouring or mixing.

– Copious washing out of the eyes by running tap water for at least 10 min: this should start as soon as possible. At the working place the contents of eye bottles filled with 2% sodium bicarbonate may be squeezed into the eyes at the very first moment: washing out with tap water should always follow.

– Never apply ointment or oil in the eyes.

– The polluted skin should also be copiously rinsed with tap water; at first pastes should be removed with an acetone–alcohol mixture.

– Sound hygiene is essential.

– Organic peroxides should be stored in glass or polyethylene containers protected against sunlight and dust.

– Fires should be extinguished with carbon tetrachloride, foam or carbon dioxide, not with water (Hess 1959).

REFERENCES

Chemical Safety Data Sheet SD-81. Benzoyl peroxide. *Manufact. Chemists' Assoc.*, Washington, 1960.

FLOYD, E. P. and H. E. STOKINGER, Toxicity studies of certain organic peroxides and hydroperoxides. *Am. Ind. Hyg. Assoc. J.*, 19 (1958) 205.

GROSFELD, J. C. M., *Onderzoekingen over het ontstaan van eczeem bij bakkers*, Thesis, Amsterdam, 1951.

HESS, W., Schutzmassnahmen bei der Verarbeitung von Niederdruckhärzen. *Schweiz. Bl. Arbeitssicherheit*, No. 22 (1959).

HORGAN, V. J., J. S. L. PHILPOT, B. W. PORTER and D. B. ROODYN, Toxicity of auto-oxidized squalene and linoleic acid, and of simpler peroxides, in relation to toxicity of radiation. *Biochem. J.*, 67 (1957) 551.

KAYANOVITCH, V. A., S. M. KAVALEROVA and S. A. TROITSKY, Problems of occupational hygiene and health conditions of operators engaged in the production of benzoyl peroxide. *Gigiena Truda i Prof. Zabolevaniya*, 6/1 (1962) 46.

KEY, M. M., V. B. PERONE and D. J. BIRMINGHAM, Patch testing in dermatitis from the newer resins. *J. Occupational Med.*, 3 (1961) 362.

KÜCHLE, H. J., Untersuchungen über die augenschädigende Wirkung organischer Peroxyde. *Zbl. Arbeitsmed.*, 8 (1958) 25.

MALTEN, K. E., *Beroepsekzeem bij het verwerken van kunststoffen*, Thesis, Amsterdam, 1956.

REES, G. P. VAN and B. A. BIJNSDORP, Unpublished investigation. Leiden, 1958.

17

Other auxiliary substances

STABILIZERS

Physico-chemical properties, application

Stabilizers are added to prevent degradation of the plastics, particularly in regard to ageing and thermal decomposition. The most important groups are (Lefaux 1952, 1961):
– Metal soaps, particularly from Pb, Cd, Ba, Sr, Sn.
– Metal salts, particularly from Pb, Mg, Na.
– Organic metal compounds, particularly from Sn.
– Internal oxides, particularly ethylene oxide, butylene oxide, epoxy resins.

The biologic properties of these compounds have been studied especially for undesirable effects when used in food packings. Some of the agents mentioned above, however, should also be discussed in view of their industrial-hygienic consequences.

Toxicology and dermatology

Lead compounds

These compounds are added as stabilizers and as pigments, for instance in PVC. Mixing occurs in a dry state: the concentrations in air easily exceed the MAC (0.1 mg Pb/m^3). Only by introduction of elaborate hygienic measures (ventilation; use of paste instead of powder; weighing in plastic bags, which were mixed as such through the polymer), Goss *et al.* (1953) could bring down the lead concentration in the urine of exposed workers to reasonable levels. The often used lead soaps, Pb stearate and Pb laureate, are very light; the dust therefore settles slowly. According to Guerdjikoff *et al.* (1958, 1959), this was a very important factor in the occurrence of lead poisoning in workers producing PVC cables, to which 3–6% Pb stearate had to be added. Zannini *et al.* (1961) reported one case of chronic poisoning and some signs of increased Pb uptake in 9 other workers when adding Pb stearate to PVC in badly ventilated surroundings. Similar experiences were mentioned by Sassi *et al.* (1961).

Cadmium compounds

These agents also are used as stabilizers and pigments, for instance in PVC. Industrial hygienic consequences have not been reported from the plastics industry.

Tin compounds

Many organic tin compounds are being added to PVC. Their toxicity is well known, but no difficulties have yet been reported from the plastics industry. Workers handling them should be under strict control. The oral toxicity of the compounds decreases with increasing length of the alkyl groups; di-*n*-octyltin possesses a slight toxicity (LD_{50}-oral for rats is 5–6 g/kg). Tetraethyltin and tetramethyltin are broken down to the very toxic trialkyl compounds (Barnes *et al.* 1958; Klimmer *et al.* 1960). Percutaneous resorption is possible (Elsea *et al.* 1958; Cruickshank 1960; Hofmann 1961). In animal experiments certain compounds proved to be greatly irritating to the skin and mucosae. During heat-processing unpleasant fumes were released. A stabilized aqueous eluate from fabricated PVC foil irritated the mucosae, especially when the stabilizer contained mercaptan bound sulfur (Pokorny 1961). Irritation of the skin and the occurrence of follicular dermatitis round the wrists were reported in workers handling triphenyltin compounds (Docter 1962).

Alkene oxides

The toxicity of ethylene oxide has extensively been studied by Hollingworth *et al.* (1956). Irritation of the air passages and damage of the lungs were observed in rats, mice, guinea pigs, rabbits and monkeys when exposed to 204 p.p.m., 7 h per day, 5 days per week; in rats and guinea pigs alterations in liver, kidney, adrenals and testes were reported; in rats, rabbits and monkeys a reversible disturbance of the nervous system occurred. Guinea pigs, rabbits and monkeys tolerated exposure to 113 p.p.m. during 6–7 months, rats and mice 49 p.p.m. for the same period. The authors proposed a MAC of 50 p.p.m. = 90 mg/m^3, which has been accepted by the A.C.G.I.H. (1962). In human beings exposed to high concentrations, the authors observed irritation of the mucosae of eyes and air passages, nausea, vomiting, dyspnoea, cyanosis, drowsiness, asthenia, incoordination, lymphocytosis, deviations in the ECG and excretion of bile pigments. The odour threshold rises during exposure, the warning effect therefore disappears. Exposure of the skin to aqueous solutions may cause serious burns, sometimes appearing only after several hours. The pure anhydride does not irritate the dry skin. After repeated application Sexton *et al.* (1949, 1950) saw skin sensitization in 3 out of 8 subjects tested.

Measures for prevention and first aid were given in the *Hygienic Guide* (1958) and *Chem. Safety Data Sheet* SD-38 (1951).

Propylene oxide has similar properties, but the experimental toxicity is about 1/3 compared with ethylene oxide (Hollingworth *et al.* 1956); A.C.G.I.H. (1962) suggested a MAC of 100 p.p.m. = 240 mg/cm^3. The MAC for butylene oxide S (mixture of three isomers) is supposed to be below 400 p.p.m. (Dow 1958).

CATALYSTS AND ACCELERATORS

Physico-chemical properties, application

Many compounds may be used as catalysts. The most important are:

– organic peroxides, non-genuine catalysts for polymerization reactions (see Chapter 16, p. 211),
– Ziegler–Natta catalysts, organic metal compounds for the polymerization of low-pressure polyethylene, usually aluminium–alkyl compounds,
– Boron compounds for polymerization of epoxy resins and polystyrene,
– simple compounds, mostly alkalies and acids, for polycondensation reactions.

Some catalytic reactions may be accelerated by a group of other compounds: accelerators. As such, cobalt soaps and dimethylaniline are used (see p. 76).

Toxicology and dermatology

Aluminium–alkyl compounds

Aluminium trimethyl and aluminium triethyl are very aggressive compounds. They are highly explosive in the presence of air, water or alcohol. By reaction with H_2O the corresponding alkane and $Al(OH)_3$ are formed, accompanied by the production of much smoke and heat; $Al(OH)_3$ is decomposed into Al_2O_3 and H_2O forming a white fog. If the compounds also contain Cl, HCl is produced in addition. The compounds mentioned above cause very painful, slowly healing burns of the skin. Smyth *et al.* (1957) could not produce any burns on rabbits' skin by application of 5, 10 or 20 % aluminium triisobutyl, but a 40 % solution was aggressive. Harris (1959), however, observed an accidental burn caused by a 20 % solution of an aluminium–alkyl compound. Exposure to 67 p.p.m. aluminium chloride-diisobutyl for 1 h caused fatal lung haemorrhages in 2 out of 6 rats; the vapours of aluminium triisobutyl were somewhat less aggressive. Because the vapours of aluminium–alkyl compounds are white and have a strong musty odour, their presence is perceptible at low concentrations. Accidentally exposed workers should be medically examined, particularly in regard to their lungs and bronchi. Knap *et al.* (1957) also reported the occurrence of metal-fume fever.

Technical and hygienic preventive measures have been extensively reviewed by Knap *et al.* (1957) and by Kröger (1960). In handling these compounds, the rule of keeping them under a blanket of an inert gas (N_2, Argon) should be strictly observed.

Boron trifluoride

(BF_3) is used in the polyaddition of epoxy resins (see p. 113), whereas decaborane ($B_{10}H_{14}$) promotes the polymerization of styrene. The boron hydrides (= boranes) are very toxic compounds: decaborane and pentaborane particularly affect the nervous system, diborane more specifically attacks lung and kidney. The following MAC values are proposed: 0.05 p.p.m., 0.01 p.p.m., 0.1 p.p.m. respectively (A.C.G.I.H. 1962; Browning 1961).

FOAMING AGENTS

Physico-chemical properties, application

Several types of plastics may be transformed into foam plastics, either in the polymer phase, or in an intermediate, non-cured phase. Two types of foam may be distinguished:

– *non-genuine foam:* to a highly viscose plastic, foaming agents are added, which produce gas bubbles *in situ* by means of a chemical reaction, an increase in temperature or a lowering in pressure. Closed bubbles are formed. Well-known foaming agents are: sodium carbonate, sodium nitrite, hydrogen peroxide, azoisobutyronitrile. Sometimes a gas is formed as by-product of the polycondensation reaction itself: CO_2 in isocyanates (see p. 87).

– *genuine foam:* a gas is introduced into a low viscosity plastic; pores connect the bubbles. One applies for instance air, CO_2, freons, methyl chloride.

Some of the foaming agents mentioned above have caused considerable difficulties in industry.

Toxicology and dermatology

Azoisobutyronitrile (= Porophor N)

releases at 190 °C nitrogen gas and a certain amount of tetramethylsuccinic-dinitrile. This substance, therefore, is produced within the resin; it cannot be avoided that the recently prepared foam should still contain this very toxic compound. It proved to be a strong convulsant; oral uptake of 25 mg/kg or exposure to 60 p.p.m. for 2–3 h or 6 p.p.m. for 30 h was lethal for rats (Spolyar, 1948). According to Hecht *et al.* (1956/1957) the oral LD_{50} for rats and mice was 30 mg/kg and 17.5–25 mg/kg respectively, whereas the LD_{50}-intraperitoneal was 17.5 mg/kg for rat. Mice died when exposed to 158 mg/m^3 for 164 min, or to 125 mg/m^3 for 200 min. Phenobarbital sodium was a good antidote. A cumulative effect did not occur. Recently prepared PVC foam still released during several days emanations lethal for mice. Application of pure powder to the skin of 6 human subjects for 24 h did not yield any abnormalities.

Reinl (1957) reported 5 cases with convulsions and coma from industries which produced or processed foam plastics. In 16 exposed subjects he noted headache (12 cases), disturbance of equilibrium (5), foamy sialorrhoea (7), nausea (7). Sometimes a hyperkinetic syndrome occurred. Physical examination did not reveal any pathology. All symptoms quickly disappeared after interruption of work; chronic intoxication was not established. Quooss (1959) mentioned 'shooting' frontal headache, drowsiness, anorexia, distended abdomen, nausea, asthenia, sleep disturbances, vertigo, vomiting, flatulence (in this order of decreasing frequency) in 13 workers (mostly female) within 8 weeks of exposure in a workshop producing life-jackets. Less serious symptoms were observed in workers making coverings for furniture or floating bodies for nets. Quooss proposed some preventive measures: use of sharp saws, prohibition of handling recently cut foams, rotation of workers. The most valid measure however proved to be use of

References p. 227

other foaming agents; in recent years most manufacturers have changed over to less noxious substances. Extra caution is necessary when foam plastics, made according to the procedure discussed above, are involved in accidental fires.

Malten (1956) found no skin sensitizations in about 15 workers engaged in sawing Vinicel (PVC-foam sheats made with Porophor-N).

Methyl chloride = monochloromethane

CH_3Cl is a well-known toxic substance. In addition to application as a refrigerant, it has also been used as foaming agent. The toxicity is considerable: after an initial narcosis, various signs of intoxication may occur as 'second disease': disturbances of nervous system, liver and kidney, anaemia. A MAC of 100 p.p.m. = 210 mg/m^3 is proposed by A.C.G.I.H. (1962). In a small workshop using styrofoam (polystyrene) as insulating layer in refrigerators one fatal case occurred, while two workers became seriously ill due to the release of methyl chloride in sawing operations (Kentucky State Dept. of Health 1959).

ANTIOXIDANTS

Physico-chemical properties, application

Antioxidants are added to obviate the effect of O_2. Some representatives are:

- phenols: bisphenol, di-*tert*.-butylmethylphenol.
- amines: *p*-phenylenediamine, hexamethylenetetramine.
- oximes.

Toxicology and dermatology

The hazard of the phenols is small. For bisphenol, see p. 108. The experimental toxicity of di-*tert*.-butylmethylphenol has been studied by Deichmann *et al*. (1955); the compound was considered relatively harmless.

p-Phenylenediamine is a well-known sensitizer for skin and respiratory tract. For hexamethylene tetramine, see p. 47.

The oximes *n*-butyraldoxime and ketoxime are applied as anti-skinning compounds in paints and inks. Only in high exposures they may give rise to a peculiar 'antabus' effect. Lewis *et al.* (1956) observed red face and eyes, dyspnoea, palpitations, tachycardia and drowsiness in a printing shop only in workers who took alcohol after working time. Chronic effects were not established. The oximes probably impeded the oxidation of alcohols; the acetic aldehyde level in the blood had considerably increased. After lowering concentration of the oximes in the inks, and better ventilation, the symptoms of intoxication disappeared.

PLASTICIZERS

Physico-chemical properties, application

Plasticizers act as 'heavy solvents' for plastics: they decrease the attractive forces between the polymer molecules, and therefore increase mouldability. The vapour pressure is minimal, the boiling point is high. The number of plasticizers which are applied, is legion. They may be added in large amounts to thermoplastic resins, sometimes up to 60% of the total weight.

Some well-known groups of plasticizers are:
- phthalates, see p. 64.
- phosphoric acid esters
- epoxy compounds, see Chapter 9, p. 118
- chlorinated paraffins
- anthracene oils
- glycols and glycol derivatives.

Toxicology and dermatology

The industrial hazard for inhalation is negligible. Extensive experimental investigations in regard to oral toxicity have, however, been carried out, considering the public health implications. These toxicity data have been reviewed by Lefaux (1952, 1960), Mallette *et al.* (1952), McCormick *et al.* (1954).

Hardly any industrial–hygienic consequences have been reported. Caution is advised in handling tri-orthocresyl phosphate which possesses a specific toxicity to the nervous system, and chlorinated paraffins which may cause acneiform dermatitis, anaemia and liver disease.

Cagianut (1954) reported an intoxication by oral uptake of one teaspoonful of dibutyl phthalate. Within 48 h the worker suffered from bilateral keratitis and showed albumen and erythrocytes in urine; recovery was complete within 2 weeks. Sutton *et al.* (1960) examined workers exposed to vapour, mist and dust of triphenyl phosphate (average 3.5 mg/m^3). A decrease of cholinesterases in erythrocytes occurred; percutaneous resorption was not established, in sharp contrast to tri-orthocresyl phosphate.

Trichloroethyl phosphate presumably releases toxic vapours of ethylene chloride and ethylene chlorohydrin when heated above 200°; extra ventilation is necessary (Ehrlicher 1962).

Dermatologic data concerning plasticizers are sparse. From a summary given by Wilson *et al.* (1954) we cite the following items: Dibutyl phthalate is a mild primary skin irritant; dioctyl phthalate has a moderate skin irritating effect, but it does not act as a sensitizer when tested as a plasticizer in vinyl film. Flexol 8N8 (N,N-di-β-(2-ethylhexyl)-ethyl-2-ethylhexylamide) and Paraplex G25, resp. G40 proved to be severe skin irritants and showed moderate sensitizing effect on the skin. Moreover diethylene glycol dicaproate, methylacetyl ricinoleate, and monotoluyldiphenyl phosphate (= Sancticizer 140) are reported to have a moderate skin-sensitizing capacity.

In 12 patients with contact hypersensitivity to Araldit D-epoxy resin, Malten (1956) observed in 4 cases a positive patch test to ethyldiglycol. A positive patch test to dioctyl phthalate was only seen once in 13 epoxy resin-positive patients, dibutyl phthalate provoked no reaction in any of them.

Fregert *et al.* (1963) recently reported contact hypersensitivity to epoxy resins used as plasticizers and stabilizers in polyvinyl chloride (PVC) resins used in household articles (PVC handbag, PVC chamberpot, necklace of surface-treated beads). Such use of a rather strong sensitizer should be stopped immediately.

REFERENCES

American Conference Governmental Industrial Hygienists, *Threshold Limit Values*, Detroit, Michigan, 1962.

BARNES, J. M. and H. B. STONER, Toxic properties of some di-alkyl and tri-alkyl tin salts. *Brit. J. Ind. Med.*, 15 (1958) 15.

BROWNING, E., *Toxicity of Industrial Metals*, Butterworths, London, 1961.

CAGIANUT, B., Keratitis erosiva und Nephritis toxica nach Einnahme von Dibutylphthalat. *Schweiz. Med. Wochschr.*, 84 (1954) 1243. Ref.: HARRIS, 1959.

Chemical Safety Data Sheet SD-38. *Ethylene Oxide*, Manufact. Chemists' Assoc., Washington, 1951.

CRUICKSHANK, C. N. D., The use of tissue cultures for toxicity tests. *Trans. Assoc. Ind. Med. Officers*, 10 (1960) 94.

DEICHMANN, W. B., J. J. CLEMMER, R. RAKOCZY and J. BIANCHINE, Toxicity of di-tertiary butylmethylphenol. *Arch. Ind. Health*, 11 (1955) 93.

DOCTER, H. J., Organische tinverbindingen. *Tijdschr. Soc. Geneesk.*, 40 (1962) 587.

Dow Chemical Company, *Butylene Oxides*, 1958.

EHRLICHER, H., Arbeitsmedizinische Fragen auf dem Kunststoffgebiet. *Kongress f. Arbeitsschutz und Arbeitsmedizin 1961*, Steinkopff, Darmstadt, 1962.

ELSEA, J. R. and O. E. PAYNTER, Toxicological studies on bis(tri-*n*-butyltin) oxide. *Arch. Ind. Health*, 18 (1958) 214.

FREGERT, S. and H. RORSMAN, Hypersensitivity to epoxy resins used as plasticizers and stabilizers in polyvinylchloride (PVC) resins. *Acta Dermato-Venereol. (Stockh.)*, 43 (1963) 10.

Goss, A. E. and A. M. Ross, Effective control of lead dust in the manufacture of vinyl plastics. *Am. Ind. Hyg. Assoc. Quart.*, 14 (1953) 41.

Guerdjikoff, C., De quelques risques saturnins peu connus du corps médical. *Z. Präv.-Med.*, 4 (1959) 292.

Guerdjikoff, C. and P. Desbaumes, L'intoxication professionnelle par le stéarate de plomb. *Rev. Méd. Suisse Rom.*, 78 (1958) 320. Ref.: *Zbl. Arbeitsmed.*, 11 (1961) 44.

Harris, D. K., Some hazards in the manufacture and use of plastics. *Brit. J. Ind. Med.*, 16 (1959) 221.

Hecht, G. and H. Kimmerle, Toxikologische Untersuchungen über Tetramethylbernsteinsäuredinitril. Unpublished investigations, 1956–1957. Ref.: Reinl, 1957.

Hofmann, H. T., Zur Frage der Gesundheitsgefährdung durch moderne Kunststoffe und ihre Lösungsmittel. *Zbl. Arbeitsmed.*, 11 (1961) 240.

Hollingworth, R. L., V. K. Rowe, F. Oyen, D. D. McCollister and H. C. Spencer, Toxicity of ethylene oxide determined on experimental animals. *Arch. Ind. Health*, 13 (1956) 217.

Hygienic Guide. Ethylene oxide. *Am. Ind. Hyg. Assoc. J.*, 19 (1958) 528.

Kentucky State Department of Health, Methyl chloride intoxication. *Publ. Health Rept. (U.S.)*, 74 (1959) 683.

Klimmer, O. R. and J. U. Nibel, Experimentelle Untersuchungen zur Frage der Toxicität einiger Stabilisatoren in Kunststoffen aus P.V.C. *Arzneimittel-Forsch.*, 10 (1960) 44.

Knap, J. E., R. E. Leech, A. J. Reid and U. S. Tamplin, Safe handling of alkyl–aluminium compounds. *Ind. Eng. Chem.*, 49 (1957) 874.

Kröger, J., Sicherheitsmassnahmen beim Umgang mit Aluminium–alkylverbindungen. *Zbl. Arbeitsmed.*, 10 (1960) 101.

Lefaux, R., *Toxicologie des Matières Plastiques et des Composés Macromoléculaires*, Masson, Paris, 1952.

Lefaux, R., Propriétés physiologiques et toxicologie des plastifiants. *Pensées Plastiques*, 7 (1960) 23.

Lefaux, R., Propriétés physiologiques et toxicologie des stabilisants pour polymères vinyliques. *Plastiques Inform.*, 12 (1961) 1, 4, 5 and 10.

Lewis, W. and L. Schwartz, The occupational disease no one talked about. *Arch. Ind. Health*, 13 (1956) 628.

McCormick, W. E. and R. H. Wilson, Toxicology of plastics. *Proc. XIth Intern. Congr. Occupational Health, Atti, Naples*, 1954, p. 107.

Mallette, F. S. and E. von Haam, Studies on the toxicity and skin effects of compounds used in the rubber and plastic industries. II. Plasticizers. *Arch. Ind. Health*, 6 (1952) 231.

Malten, K. E., *Beroepsekzeem bij het verwerken van kunststoffen*, Thesis, Amsterdam, 1956.

Oettel, H., Gesundheitsgefährdung durch Kunststoffe. *Arch. Exptl. Pathol. Pharmakol.*, 232 (1958) 77.

Pokorny, F. Toxicity of some new organo-tin stabilizers in the plastic industry. *Pracovni Lékar.*, 13 (1961) 439. Ref.: *CIS Docum., Domi*, 168–1962.

Quooss, H., *Gesundheitsgefahren in der Kunststoffindustrie*, Barth, Leipzig, 1959.

Reinl, W., Erkrankungen durch Tetramethylbernsteinsäuredinitril bei der Schaumstoffherstellung. *Arch. Toxikol.*, 16 (1957) 367.

Sassi, C., M. Finulli and C. Nava, Saturnism in the processing of lead stearate. *Med. Lavoro*, 52 (1961) 1958. Ref.: *Bull. Hyg.*, 37 (1962) 934.

Sexton, R. J. and E. V. Henson, Dermatological injuries by ethylene oxide. *J. Ind. Hyg.*, 31 (1949) 297.

Sexton, R. J. and E. V. Henson, Experimental ethylene oxide human skin injuries. *Arch. Ind. Health*, 2 (1950) 549.

Smyth, H. F. and C. P. Carpenter, Unpublished reports. Chemical hygiene fellowship, Mellon Institute. Ref.: Knap *et al.*, 1957.

Spolyar, L. W., Indiana chemist's report on toxicity of product of Porofor N. *Ind. Hyg. Newsletter*, 8 (1948) 3. Ref.: Oettel (1957).

Sutton, W. L., C. J. Terhaar, F. A. Miller, R. F. Scherberger, E. C. Riley, R. L. Roudabush and D. W. Fassett, Studies on the industrial hygiene and toxicology of triphenyl phosphate. *Arch. Environ. Health*, 1 (1960) 33.

Wilson, R. H. and W. E. McCormick, Toxicology of plastics and rubbers – plastomers and monomers. *Ind. Med. Surg.*, 23 (1954) 479.

Zannini, D. and F. Lombardi, Intoxication due à l'usage des stabilisateurs contenant des sels de plomb pour matières plastiques. *Lavoro umano*, 13 (1961) 145. Ref.: *Arch. Maladies Profess.*, 23 (1962) 178.

18

Prevention of occupational dermatoses in working-up plastics

DIAGNOSIS

For the prevention of occupational dermatoses the diagnosis is of first and utmost importance. An adequate diagnosis must be regarded as a keystone for prevention.

It depends entirely on the clinical picture in what way the investigation should be made, *e.g.* in an oil-acne patient one need not look for a sensitizer; in a dyshydrosis-patient (as one of many possibilities) inhalation of a sensitizer is more likely to be the causative mechanism than direct skin contact with a sensitizing substance. However, it may be remembered from Chapter 4 dealing with occupational dermatoses that hybrids between toxic dermatitis and contact allergic eczema frequently occur. In toxic dermatitis, contact eczema and their hybrids, one's thoughts do not go into any particular direction because simply *all* substances in the environment of the worker must be suspected, unless the localization (in sporadic cases) makes it possible to restrict the range of suspected substances to a few.

The investigator should thus be provided with every possible *information* concerning substances, methods and working habits, in order to gain a clear view over all possibilities. If information as to the exact composition of mixtures marketed under fancy names is lacking, he should have the opportunity to investigate them thoroughly before they are introduced on a large scale. Generally speaking, the right place for a medical officer is next to the construction engineer and next to the chemist, the production designer and the architect of the workshop. Their cooperation will bring about an alertness, due to which dangers may be recognized before they lead to catastrophes.

Unfortunately the medical tools of investigation are still scarce. In the case of dermatitis one seldom passes the stage of suspecting a number of primary irritants from the environment, but in the case of contact eczema the exact cause may be found through patch-testing with *all* possible contactants, provided this is done with a safe concentration in a safe solvent in a quiet phase of the patient's illness. This is the only manner to spot polysensitizations which, if undetected, might puzzle the management concerned in finding a new job assignment for a sensitized worker.

PREVENTIVE MEASURES

If, in a certain work, primary skin irritation or sensitization frequently occur, the possibility of *substituting* a less harmful substance for the incriminated one should be seriously considered (remember the M.I.P.-hardeners for epoxy resins and the mixtures of peroxides with plasticizers for unsaturated polyesters).

If a certain type of work has to be repeated several times, if a certain product has to be made in series, if during working up, the pieces can be fixed in a certain position, then the possibility of *mechanizing* the process can be suggested. Frequently, this requires less skin contact with chemicals in their active state. Thus the working up of epoxy resins in factories making large series of simple, small electrical appliances need not be a grave problem.

The *separation* of the hazardous phase of the processing cycle from the normal process may have obvious advantages. Thus in building hat racks, the working up of epoxy resins should be done separately, at a different time and place, and by workers who do not handle polyester resins (see Chapter 7). In repairing shoes, the cobbler should first prepare all shoes up to the glueing phase. Then, at a certain time scheduled for the job, he should change his apron and tools and, seated in a more or less separated part of his workshop, he should dispatch all the glueing work in one tour. In this way, secondary contamination through transfer of the noxious substance adhering to the gloves and tools is checked; besides, skin contact with the potential sensitizers in the adhesive is limited to a short time of the day, instead of being spread over the whole working time, and contamination is not dispersed through the entire workshop by the tools (see p. 49).

If possible, the handling of primary toxic agents should be separated from handling sensitizers. Thus, in laminating unsaturated polyesters with glass-fibre cloth, the cutting of the cloth to the appropriate shape should be done by a worker who does not touch the liquid resin mixture.

Occupational hygienic measures must be taken in all events in which the spreading of noxious agents can be stopped at the sites of generation or the duration of contamination can be shortened. For instance:

– In cutting glass-fibre cloth, the table leaf should be furnished with exhaust devices (slits) along the elevated rims.

– Batch mixing of resins and hardeners or accelerators may give rise to unusual generation of vapours due to a rise in temperature of the mixture. These vapours may be harmful (amines, peroxides, phthalic acid anhydrides) and, therefore, this work should be done in a separated area, by a few workers, under a ventilated hood.

– Quantities of the resin mixtures appropriate to fulfill a certain requirement should be distributed in paper cups, which should be thrown away after use.

– If large areas are to be provided with an epoxy resin, DTA or TTA hardener mixture, this should be done under exhaust ventilation. The piece of work must be situated between the worker and the mouth of the flexible pipe exhaust.

– If the rims of press goods are sticky, this means that the curing

out has not yet been completed at these sites. They should be allowed to dry before the goods are machined further.
– Grinding, sawing, drilling or polishing moulded laminates should be done under local exhaust ventilation to remove all glass-fibre dust from the breathing area and minimize skin contact.
– In the case of epoxy resins, this measure may be appropriate to prevent untoward effects as described by Bourne (1956) in a sensitized worker who reacted with generalized paresthesia, pruritis, edema, drowsiness and diarrhoea after short exposures in a laboratory where the resin was being machined.
– The tables can be kept clean by using heavy paper sheets that are from time to time discarded.
– The tools should be thoroughly cleaned with an excess of suitable solvent after each shift by a worker assigned specially for this duty, who wears gloves during work. The tools should be preferably soaked in a solvent bath to dissolve the partly cured resin contamination, and then cleaned one by one with cotton wool wetted with the solvent, that is discarded after use.
– A certain time should be assigned for clean-up prior to breaks and closing time.
– Full attention should be paid to the *working method.* In applying the resin mixtures it is often possible to use spatules or brushes with a long handle instead of the bare hands. When small localized droplets of resin mixture are to be applied on a certain site of the piece of work, this may sometimes be done with the help of a movable air-pressure gun instead of a brush which may drip on the way from storage tin to object.
– When glass-fibre epoxy laminates must be fastened to aluminium honeycomb, we have observed that the workers followed a special method which may have a wider field of application. The working table was covered by a plastic foil of appropriate shape, upon which the precut fibre-glass cloth was applied alternately with the resin mixture. The latter was rubbed in with a large spatule. When a certain thickness of the lami-

References p. 236

nate was reached the whole laminate together with the foil backing was moved from the table to the honeycomb, which was set up in almost vertical position. The wet laminate was pressed against the honeycomb with the fingers; these became, however, not soiled thanks to the plastic foil backing (the table side of which was not contaminated with the resin mixture). The workers should be encouraged to invent and develop work methods which combine efficiency with cleanliness.

With respect to *selection* it should be remembered that case histories, if correctly interpreted, may contain information about former contact sensitizations. Pre-employment patch-testing is of no use and should therefore be avoided (Lauer 1956). Further criteria for selection may be to employ dark-haired workers (Grandjean 1957) whose skin is not dry and scaly. Workers with non-occupational skin ailments should not be employed for this chemical work. Above all, the prospective worker should have a clean and tidy appearance, the intelligence to understand and fulfill particular working requirements and the willingness to observe certain precautionary measures, especially cleanliness.

We concur with the opinion of Hine *et al.* (1958) that one of the most important measures for combating dermatitis from (epoxy) resins is the practice of *good personal hygiene:*

– Aprons and sleeves can be worn, which may be rubbed in with a parting compound. To wear gloves is seldom possible. These articles must be made of materials resisting the chemicals used. Schwartz *et al.* (1940) reported on a testing device.

– Barrier creams may be used if contamination is inevitable; care must be taken that the cream chosen protects, against all components involved. Thus Kerodex BW2 or BD6 or Rosalex 9 may prove effective against amine hardeners but not against the epoxy resins, the reverse was true for silicones. At the start of every working period a good layer of the cream must be rubbed in until it has dried. Then a second layer is rubbed in which is thinner than the first.

– To remove accidental spills, a resin-removing cream should be at hand for prompt application, but if the resin–hardener mixture has been in contact with the skin for only a short time, soap and water suffice.
– Neutral or acid soaps are to be preferred if the substances handled are strongly alkaline. The resin–hardener mixture should not be allowed to cure out on the skin and then be picked off, because in doing so one removes the upper layer of the epidermis and thus enables the chemicals to penetrate into lower layers of the skin at the next contamination (Bourne *et al.* 1959).
– Personally we are inclined to advise cleansing only the contaminated area of the skin with a piece of cotton wool moistened with a suitable solvent (acetone, methyl ethyl ketone), which must be thrown away after use; this should be repeated once or twice. The solvent is provided from a dispenser with a foot pedal. The skin may then be rinsed with water and acid soap, dried with a paper towel and rubbed in with a cream containing water and a non-mineral grease.
– In working with volatile substances it may be useful to apply a barrier cream on the face and the neck, because parts of the skin in these areas are easily penetrated.
– It must be kept in mind that thorough cleansing of the hands before using lavatories is necessary for the same reason.
– Clean-up rags should be replaced by disposable paper towels, because rags not only spread the contamination over a larger area but also they never clean effectively.

All bottles and tins containing chemicals should be *labelled* throughout the factory so that, in case of an accident, there should be no doubt as to which chemical was responsible for it. The workers should be aware of the hazards that the chemicals they handle involve. It should be pointed out to them that they might become sensitized without premonitory signs, even if the incriminated substance has been handled for months or years without untoward experience. On the other hand, one must take care not to alarm the workers. This may be avoided by

References p. 236

comparing sensitizing materials from the plastics industries with household substances, say turpentine or nickel.

– The workers should be told how to keep their skin in good condition. They should report at the medical ward even with minor skin involvements and injuries.

Frequent supervisory *instruction* at varying moments of the working hours is indispensable to instal and maintain good working habits.

To summarize: preventive measures must be taken within the scope of the actual relationship between the handled substance and the worker. It is possible to tackle the problem of *sound hygienic measures* on various levels. Measures taken in direct relation to the substance will show a lasting result: substitution, mechanization, segregation, occupational hygienic measures. The success of measures concerning the workers' attitude depends on human factors. Among such may be included: working methods, selection, personal hygiene, instruction and supervision. All possibilities discussed above to lessen skin contact with chemicals should be considered, in order to create optimal working conditions.

REFERENCES

BOURNE, L. B., Medical problems associated with epi-oxide-resins. *Trans. Assoc. Ind. Med. Officers*, 6 (1956) 94.

BOURNE, L.B., F.J.M. MILNER and K.B. ALBERMAN, Health problems of epoxy resins and amine-curing agents. *Brit. J. Ind. Med.*, 16 (1959) 81.

GRANDJEAN, E., The danger of dermatoses due to coldsetting ethoxyline resins (epoxide resins). *Brit. J. Ind. Med.*, 14 (1957) 1.

LAUER, D. J., Preplacement patch tests. *Penn. Med. J.*, 59 (1956) 25.

HINE, C. H., J. K. KODAMA, H. H. ANDERSON, D. W. SIMONSON and J. S. WELLINGTON, The toxicology of epoxy resins. *Arch. Ind. Health*, 17 (1958) 129.

SCHWARTZ, L., L. H. WARREN and F. H. GOLDMAN, Clothing for protection against occupational skin irritants. *Public Health Rept. (U.S.)*, 55 (1940) 1158.

List of patch-testing concentrations

of a number of substances encountered in the field of plastics

WARNING

1. The manufacturers of the ingredients (mixtures) listed below might alter the composition of their product without notice. Although the solvents and concentrations listed seemed appropriate at the time of investigation to determine whether or not a patient was contact-hypersensitive, this might not be true in the future, due to possible alterations in composition.
2. These patch-testing concentrations were found to be appropriate for 24-h patch-testing exposures. Longer exposures under patch-testing conditions (technique described in Chapter 4) may give untoward effects, such as severe local and possibly focal reactions.
3. As a number of solvents are more or less volatile, it is of utmost importance to use freshly prepared solutions.
4. If the solvent is changed for any reason, the patch-testing concentration should be adjusted; for instance, 5% triethylenetetramine in alcohol is appropriate, the same concentration in water is far too high, due to the high degree of alkalinity present.

If you are not quite *sure*, try the solution on your own skin first. The investigator, not the patient, should be the first testing rabbit!

Compound		*Concentration in solvent*
AC 444 C 21	(di-isocyanate system)	10% methyl ethyl ketone
AC 444 C 21 hardener	(di-isocyanate system)	10% ethyl acetate
AC 444 C 21 thinner	(di-isocyanate system)	10% ethyl acetate
acrylate emulsion		60% aqua
acryl inner lacquer 6172		10% acetone
acrylonitrile		5% amyl alcohol
adipic acid		100%
Aerodux 185 (Aeroresearch)		40% acetone
Aerodux hardener HPR 150		100%
Aerolite 306		50% alcohol aqua āā
Aerolite hardener GMB		10% aqua
AGO casting resin Acrylon 617 H7		10% acetone
AGO Innengrundierung 61726		10% acetone
AGOmet E (acryl)		20% ethyl acetate
AGOmet M(acryl)		20% ethyl acetate
AGOmet hardener		10% alcohol (shake)
AGO thinner 634 A10		10% alcohol
allylglycidyl ether		2% acetone
ammonia		2% aqua
ammonium molybdate		2% aqua
ammonium vanadate		2% aqua
amyl acetate		100%
antimony trioxide		100%
Araldit 101 (epoxy resin, Ciba) (= AY 101)		70% acetone
Araldit 102 (epoxy resin, Ciba)		70% acetone
Araldit 103 (epoxy resin, Ciba) (= AY 103)		70% acetone
Araldit metal-bonding resin 121 B (epoxy resin, Ciba) (= AV 121 B)		10% acetone
Araldit metal-bonding resin 121 N (epoxy resin, Ciba) (= AV 121 N)		40% acetone (shake)
Araldit metal-bonding resin 123 B (epoxy resin, Ciba) (= AV 123 B)		30% acetone
Araldit SW 400 (epoxy resin, Ciba)		70% acetone

Compound	*Concentration in solvent*
Araldit SW 402 (epoxy resin, Ciba)	70% acetone
Araldit SW 417 (epoxy resin, Ciba)	70% acetone
Araldit 430 (epoxy resin, Ciba)	40% acetone
Araldit 431 (epoxy resin, Ciba)	40% acetone
Araldit LW 551 (epoxy resin, Ciba)	70% acetone
Araldit laminating resin 553 (epoxy resin, Ciba) (= LY 553)	40% acetone
Araldit laminating resin 556 (epoxy resin, Ciba) (= LY 556)	40% acetone
Araldit laminating hardener + resin	70% acetone
Araldit B (epoxy resin, Ciba) (= CT 200)	70% acetone
Araldit D (epoxy resin, Ciba) (= CY 230)	70% acetone
Araldit DS (epoxy resin, Ciba)	70% acetone
Araldit E (epoxy resin, Ciba) (= CY 232)	40% acetone
Araldit F (epoxy resin, Ciba) (= CY 205)	70% acetone
Araldit G (epoxy resin, Ciba)	70% acetone
Araldit M (epoxy resin, Ciba)	70% acetone
Artonex lacquer	60% acetone
Artonex hardener	10% alcohol
Artonex solvens	50% acetone
Atlas AGO hardener (acryl)	10% alcohol
Bakelite polyester SK 17449	10% acetone
Breon 599	70% aqua
Breonlatex (40% butadiene acrylonitrile emulsion)	70% ethyl acetate
BT 309 (melamine formaldehyde resin)	70% acetone
Butanox	½% alcohol
butylglycidyl ether	1% acetone

Compound	*Concentration in solvent*
cadmium stearate	100%
calcium stearate	100%
caprolactam	5% aqua
casting resin solvens 136 K 10	10% toluene ol. olivarum āā
catalyst H7	10% aqua
Cellonglue R 43-4	10% ethyl acetate
cellosolve solvens	50% aqua
Cerechloor	100%
Colorpaste Casting resin FC 41/912 R	25% acetone
copper naphthenate	10% ol. olivarum
cresylglycidyl ether	0.5% ol. olivarum
cyclohexane	40% ol. olivarum
cyclohexanol	40% ol. olivarum
cyclohexanone	50% ol. olivarum
cyclohexanone hydroperoxide	½% alcohol
cyclopentadiene	10% alcohol
decaline	40% ol. olivarum
diacetone alcohol	50% aqua
diammonium phosphate	1% aqua
dibutyl phthalate	100%
dibutyltin maleate	40% benzene ol. olivarum āā
diethylene glycol	10% aqua
diethyl ester of maleic acid*	½% alcohol
di-isocyanate system:	
AC 444 C 21	10% methyl ethyl ketone
AC 444 C 21 hardener	10% ethyl acetate
AC 444 C 21 thinner	10% ethyl acetate
dimethyl aniline	10% ol. olivarum
dimethyl ethylene urea	50% aqua
dimethylol ethylene urea	50% aqua
dimethylol triazon	50% aqua

* Patch tests should not be done with this substance as it may sensitize the patient in a 24-h epicutaneous contact (see Chapter 6, p. 66).

Compound	*Concentration in solvent*
dimethylol urea	50% aqua
dimethyl phthalate	1% aqua
2,4-dimethyl-6-*tert*.-butylphenol	10% amyl alcohol
dioctyl adipate	40% alcohol
dioctyl phthalate	100%
di-*o*-cresylolpropane	5% alcohol
diphenylamine	5% amyl alcohol
diphenylol propane	40% alcohol
EC 801	100%
EC 807	5% acetone
epichlorohydrin	1% alcohol
Epicote 828	70% acetone
ethyl acetate	100%
ethyl diglycol	40% alcohol
ethylene glycol	20% aqua
fluid foil 130 K 12	10% toluene ethyl acetate āā
formaldehyde	1% aqua
fumaric acid	100%
Grundierung G 750	10% ol. olivarum
guanidine carbonate	100%
hardener Agomet	10% alcohol (shake)
hardener Atlas Ago	10% alcohol
hardener DMP 30	2% ethyl acetate
hardener DTA	5% alcohol
hardener GMBX	1% aqua
hardener Metaflex K	10% alcohol 60%
hardener Plastoid 018 blue	5% acetone
hardener XV (Ciba)	15% alcohol
hardener SW 400 (Ciba)	20% alcohol
hardener SW 402 (Ciba)	10% alcohol
hardener SW 417 (Ciba)	5% alcohol
hardener 430 (Ciba)	10% alcohol

Compound	*Concentration in solvent*
hardener 431 (Ciba)	10% alcohol
hardener LW 551 (Ciba)	10% alcohol
hardener 553 (Ciba)	½% alcohol
hardener 901 (Ciba) (= HT 901)	0.2% ethyl acetate
hardener 902 (Ciba) (= HT 902)	0.5% ethyl acetate
hardener HY 908 (Ciba)	5% alcohol
hardener 911 (Ciba)	1% acetone
hardener 930 (Ciba) (= HY 930)	2% alcohol
hardener 931 (Ciba)	10% alcohol
hardener 951 (Ciba) (= HY 951)	5% alcohol
hardener 953 B (Ciba) (= HV 953)	10% alcohol
hardener HY 956 (Ciba)	10% alcohol
hardener 972 (Ciba)	10% alcohol
hardener AC 444 C 21 (di-isocyan. syst.)	10% ethyl acetate
hardener T 102	20% alcohol
hexachloroxylene	5% toluene ol. olivarum āā
hexamethylenetetramine	100%
Hobilon C	5% acetone
Hobilon Z (1% cobalt naphthenate in styrene)	5% alcohol
hydrazine hydrate	1% aqua
2-hydroxy-3-methylbenzylalcohol diacetate	1% amyl alcohol
Kallodent liquid } methylmethacrylate system	40% acetone
Kallodent powder } methylmethacrylate system	100%
Kerocleanse 22	5% aqua
Lamellon 6 (polyester resin Zaanchemie)	50% acetone
Lamellon 23 (polyester resin Zaanchemie)	50% acetone
Lamellon 31 (polyester resin Zaanchemie)	40% acetone

Compound	*Concentration in solvent*
Lamellon 41 (polyester resin Zaanchemie)	50 % acetone
Lamellon 51 (polyester resin Zaanchemie)	50 % methyl ethyl ketone
Lamellon 53 (polyester resin Zaanchemie)	40 % methyl ethyl ketone
Lamellon 75 (polyester resin Zaanchemie)	40 % acetone
Lamellon 237 (polyester resin Zaanchemie)	40 % acetone
Laminac 4128 (polyester resin)	40 % acetone
lead stearate	100 %
Lerocol O 3742	10 % toluene ol. olivarum āā
Lucidol C 50	1 % acetone
Lucidol paste (1 % benzoyl peroxide)	5 % acetone
Lyofix CH (melamine formaldehyde resin)	70 % acetone
maleic acid anhydride	½ % acetone
manganese naphthenate	10 % ol. olivarum
melamine formaldehyde	50 % aqua
Metaflex K hardener	10 % alcohol 60 %
1-methoxy-2-cyanomethane	5 % amyl alcohol
2-methyl cyclohexanone	1 % alcohol
2-methyl-6(dimethylaminomethyl)-phenol	5 % amyl alcohol
methylene chloride	5 % aqua
methyl ethyl ketone	100 %
methyl ethyl ketone hydroperoxide	½ % acetone
methyl glycol	50 % alcohol
methyl methacrylate liquid	5 % acetone
2-methyl-6(methoxymethyl)-phenol	10 % amyl alcohol
methyl nadic anhydride	2 % acetone
methylol melamine	35 % aqua
2-methyl-4-*tert*.-butylphenol	7 % amyl alcohol

Compound	*Concentration in solvent*
Orthofol (Teufel)	10% alcohol
Palatal KR 1144	10% acetone
Palatal P6	10% acetone
p-tert.-butyl catechol	1% acetone
p-tert.-butylphenol	30% amyl alcohol ol. olivarum āā
p-toluene sulfonyl chloride	5% aqua
p-toluidine	10% alcohol
p-tolunitrile	8% alcohol
perchloroethylene	5% acetone
phenol	3% aqua
phenol resin CKR 1634 (Union Carbide)	30% ethyl acetate
phenol resin CKR 1734 (Union Carbide)	30% ethyl acetate
phenol resin CKR 2400 (Union Carbide)	30% ethyl acetate
phthalic acid anhydride	1% alcohol
Plastoid 017	10% alcohol
Plastoid foaming agent 018 yellow	10% ol. olivarum
Plastoid hardener 018 blue	5% acetone
polyacrylamide	80% aqua
Polyamid 115	25% alcohol
polyurethane system:	
Stafoam AA 1802 RC	10% acetone
Stafoam 1802 A	10% acetone
polyvinyl acetate emulsion 55%	30% aqua
polyvinyl alcohol	25% aqua
Porofor N	10% acetone
Pressglue Footwell	10% acetone
Pressglue 1030 Helmitin	30% ethyl acetate
Primal B 15 (acryl resin emulsion)	50% aqua
propylenediamine	5% alcohol
propylene glycol	10% aqua
pyridine	30% ol. olivarum

Compound	*Concentration in solvent*
Redux K6 liquid	80% ol. olivarum
Redux powder (polyvinyl formal)	100%
Rubbolstopper A 1000	70% acetone
Santobrite (sodium pentachlorophenol)	3% alcohol
Shoe adhesive ingredients:	
cement 5739 (Boston Oberusel)	30% ethyl acetate
cement glue M 30	30% ethyl acetate
Helmitex aktiv 1024 (Heinicke)	30% ethyl acetate
Helmitin kleber 1030/1 (Heinicke)	30% ethyl acetate
Helmitin spez. kleber 1245 (Heinicke)	30% ethyl acetate
Helmitin 31120 (Heinicke)	30% ethyl acetate
Irutex S 115 (Isarchemie)	30% ethyl acetate
Isadur 438 (Isarchemie)	30% ethyl acetate
phenol-formaldehyde resin CKR 1634 (Union Carbide)	30% ethyl acetate
phenol-formaldehyde resin CKR 1734 (Union Carbide)	30% ethyl acetate
UN vulcanizing glue (Helmitin)	30% ethyl acetate
UN vulcanizing glue-hardener A	30% ethyl acetate
Vorstreichkleber (Boston Oberusel)	30% ethyl acetate
Vorstreichlösung (Heinicke)	30% ethyl acetate
Vorstreichmittel 578	30% ethyl acetate
Vulcafix C 75	30% ethyl acetate
Wakolfix 1167 B – 1167 H (Wakol)	30% ethyl acetate
Wakolfix 1422 (Wakol)	30% ethyl acetate
Wakolfix 1740 (Wakol)	30% ethyl acetate
Silicone emulsion	100%
Silicone resin SR 82	30% ethyl acetate
Simson 613	10% toluene ol. olivarum āā
Simson 1000	50% toluene ol. olivarum āā

Compound	*Concentration in solvent*
Simson hardener RF	5% alcohol
Stadoflex	50% acetone
styrene	5% alcohol
terephthaloyl chloride	5% toluene ol. olivarum āā
tetrachlorophthalic acid anhydride	1% alcohol
thinner 634 (Ago)	10% alcohol
thinner casting resin 136 K 10 (Blum)	10% toluene ol. olivarum āā
thinner M 600	30% ol. olivarum
Thiokoll LP 33 (Ciba)	30% acetone
toluene	50% ol. olivarum
triazone	50% aqua
trichloroethylene	50% ol. olivarum
tricresol	3% ol. olivarum
tricresyl phosphate	70% alcohol
2,4,6-tridimethyl-amino-methyl-phenol	2% ethyl acetate
triethylamine	10% alcohol
Trigonox K 70	½% acetone
3,4,5-trimethoxybenzyl alcohol	5% alcohol
3,4,5-trimethoxybenzyl chloride	5% alcohol
urea	10% aqua
urea formaldehyde ether	35% aqua
urea formaldehyde resin	70% acetone
Uformite (dimethylol ethylene urea)	70% acetone
Versamid 115 (Ciba)	40% ethyl acetate
Versamid 125 (Ciba)	10% toluene ol. olivarum āā
Versamid 140 (Ciba)	10% alcohol
white spirit	20% ol. olivarum
xylene	50% ol. olivarum

Subject Index

PRINTED IN THE NETHERLANDS BY
ZUID-NEDERLANDSE DRUKKERIJ N.V., 'S-HERTOGENBOSCH